A HANDBOOK OF UROLOGY
FOR STUDENTS AND
PRACTITIONERS

A
HANDBOOK OF UROLOGY
FOR STUDENTS AND
PRACTITIONERS

by

VERNON PENNELL

M.A., M.B., B.Chir., Cantab., F.R.C.S. (Eng.)

*Hon. Surgeon, and Surgeon with Charge of Urological
Department, Addenbrooke's Hospital, Cambridge;
Consulting Surgeon, Royston and District
Hospital. Fellow and Assistant Tutor,
Pembroke College, Cambridge. Fellow
of the Association of Surgeons
of Great Britain and Ireland*

CAMBRIDGE
AT THE UNIVERSITY PRESS
1936

CAMBRIDGE
UNIVERSITY PRESS

University Printing House, Cambridge CB2 8BS, United Kingdom

Cambridge University Press is part of the University of Cambridge.

It furthers the University's mission by disseminating knowledge in the pursuit of education, learning and research at the highest international levels of excellence.

www.cambridge.org
Information on this title: www.cambridge.org/9781107456341

© Cambridge University Press 1936

First published 1936
First paperback edition 2014

A catalogue record for this publication is available from the British Library

ISBN 978-1-107-45634-1 Paperback

CONTENTS

COLOURED PLATES

PREFACE

The present trend towards specialization in the diagnosis and treatment of disease, although possessing many advantages, carries with it a serious handicap from the point of view of the student in the larger teaching hospitals. Diseases of certain systems have a habit of gravitating to special hospitals. or to isolated departments in the larger general hospitals: ophthalmology, obstetrics, gynaecology, orthopaedics, and ear, nose, and throat work, are but a few examples that will occur to all. Diseases of the urinary tract have for some time past possessed their special hospitals and departments, and a knowledge of this subject is in danger of becoming relegated to post-graduate instruction, with a corresponding hiatus in the efficient clinical make-up of students and practitioners.

It is the aim of this present work to place before this large body of people a short and concise account of urinary diseases, with their method of investigation and treatment. In order to keep the size of the volume within the accepted bounds of a hand-book, rare diseases and uncommon and obsolete treatment have been rigorously pruned. Venereal disease and other infections of the genital tract have been omitted, except where their effects are more marked on the urinary than the genital system (e.g. affections of the prostate, and genito-urinary tuberculosis). Details of operative technique have been reduced to a minimum, and only those methods now most commonly employed have been described.

Of the many deficiencies of this small volume the writer is

acutely conscious, and if a certain dogmatism should have crept into the text, it represents only the considered judgment of the author, after weighing the evidence as he has heard and seen it, together with a laudable desire to avoid a still further loading of the already crowded medical curriculum.

Thanks are due to Dr C. G. L. Wolf, Honorary Biochemist to Addenbrooke's Hospital, for the section on the tests of renal efficiency described in chapter I.

V. P.

1936

Chapter I

INVESTIGATION

The urinary system consists of the kidneys, ureters, bladder and urethra, to which may be added the accessory sexual gland —the prostate—since its ills are more likely to be reflected in the urinary than in the genital system.

The investigation of any urological disease falls under the following headings:

        (1) Clinical.
        (2) Radiological.
        (3) Bacteriological.
        (4) Biochemical.

CLINICAL EXAMINATION

The clinical examination of a urological patient, although perhaps more limited, is no less important than the same investigation in patients suffering from diseases of other systems.

Unfortunately, the present-day perfection in instrument making, and the comparative ease of instrumentation on behalf of the practitioner, has led to increasing time being spent on the pure urological examination at the expense of the clinical. This is unfortunate, for, as any urologist will readily recall, essential points discovered in the clinical examination may be of greater significance than any brought out by radiology or cystoscopy.

The patient's complaint is of paramount importance and, fortunately, he is apt to come to the point with commendable briskness. Most of these patients complain of one or more prominent symptoms, e.g. frequency of micturition, pain or difficulty in passing water, incontinence, colic, haematuria, and pyuria, or abdominal tumour. It is the investigation of these leading symptoms, together with such less common ones as thirst, drowsiness, and various aches, to which the urologist must turn in making his diagnosis.

A careful history as to the inception of the complaint, its duration, or any factors influencing its severity is, of course, a *sine qua non*. The objective examination of the patient should be directed towards his general condition, particular attention being paid to the following organs and regions:

(1) **The Tongue.** In few diseases does the tongue give such a good indication of the inward condition of the patient as in certain diseases of the urinary tract. A dry, cracked tongue, associated with brown fur—often designated "parrot tongue" —is indicative of renal insufficiency and the retention in the blood of nitrogenous bodies normally excreted. Although all medical text-books make mention of a "parrot tongue" in uraemia, few stress the importance of the dry, brown or black-coated tongue, indicative of renal insufficiency and failure as an evidential point in prognosis after certain operations, or its value as a deterrent to grave operation.

(2) **Inspection and Palpation of the Abdomen.** Briefly, the flanks and the pubic region are the two areas likely to manifest evidence of disease of the urinary system. A palpable, or mobile kidney may easily be detected, and a swollen and tender one even more so. Occasionally, a much swollen and thickened ureter can be felt on the posterior abdominal wall, in thin patients, just before it crosses the pelvic brim.

Muscular rigidity, especially if unassociated with superficial tenderness, and occurring or increasing in paroxysms, is characteristic of renal and ureteric colic. Rigidity of the anterior abdominal wall, intense pain radiating from loin to groin, or testis, together with marked tenderness situated deeply in the loin, is almost diagnostic of the passage down the ureter of a renal calculus. The subsequent history of a slight haematuria, and the sudden cessation of pain, merely serve to confirm a diagnosis already made.

Palpation above the pubis may demonstrate a thickened, or abnormal bladder, while the large cystic midline swelling of a patient suffering from so-called "frequency" is characteristic of a bladder retained but overflowing. Mistakes are commonly made by students and practitioners from the nonrecognition that "frequency" may be a synonym on the part of the patient for retention and overflow. The palpation of a midline swelling, sometimes reaching from pubis to umbilicus, is—except in rare cases of markedly obese abdominal walls—of extreme simplicity, and the diagnosis of retention and overflow obvious. The passage of a catheter with the disappearance of the tumour will, of course, confirm the diagnosis.

The deep palpation of the posterior abdominal wall may bring to light abnormal masses, e.g. lymph glands, marked enlargement of kidneys or their pelves, and, rarely, ureteric calculi of large size.

The characteristics of renal swellings are well described in any text-book, but the following points are worthy of accentuation:

(a) A renal tumour, unless very large or fixed, moves up and down with respiration.

(b) It can be grasped bimanually, the fingers of one hand being placed in the loin and the flat of the other hand on the anterior abdominal wall, between which two hands the tumour can be defined and its irregularities noted.

(c) It can be "reduced" into the loin. This is diagnostic of renal tumours. Although certain swellings, which later prove to be renal in origin, may not always be entirely "reduced" into the loin, yet a lump which *can* be manipulated into this position is invariably renal in origin.

More rarely the nature of the tumour can be demonstrated. The large, smooth, cystic hydronephrosis feels quite different from the irregular, nodular swelling which has its origin in growth, or polycystic kidney.

(*d*) Renal swellings are usually resonant to percussion anteriorly—due to the presence of colon in front of them—and this characteristic in the hands of a skilled clinician will differentiate them from enlargements of liver and gall-bladder on the right side, or spleen on the left.

(3) **The Groin.** An examination of the groin and scrotum may bring to light the presence of enlarged glands, thickened cords, and abnormal conditions of testis, epididymis and vas.

The close relationship between the urinary and the genital system is well instanced in cases of tuberculosis of the bladder, and, as will be shown later, this condition is invariably secondary to some focus placed elsewhere, e.g. the kidney, or testis, and an enlarged or tender epididymis, or nodular (beaded) vas deferens, may draw the attention of the examiner to an unsuspected primary lesion.

(4) **Rectal Examination.** In no class of case is a rectal examination more necessary than in the urological.

The enlarged, or swollen prostate, palpable vesicula seminalis, and distended bladder, are easily felt. Nodules and stony hardness of the prostate—suggestive of malignant disease—variations in its contour, size and consistence, and the mobility of rectal mucous membrane, can all be detected by the examining finger, while at the same time primary rectal growths, or extensions from bladder or prostate can be felt, and any blood or slime on the finger noted. A bimanual examination may reveal changes in the bladder wall, such as extensions of growth through it to the perivesical tissues and its resultant fixity.

Less commonly, stones situated in the lower ends of the ureters are palpable, although it is uncommon to feel these in the male without the administration of an anaesthetic.

(5) **Vaginal Examination.** This is of more importance in the female than the rectal, and calculi at the lower end of the ureters can usually be felt when present and of fair size, while fixity of bladder to vagina and uterus can be determined.

(6) **Examination of the Urine.** The presence of abnormal constituents, albumen, sugar, pus, blood, bile or excessive amounts of salts (e.g. phosphates, uric acid or oxalates), together with the reaction (acid, alkaline or neutral) can readily be shown by the elementary chemical and microscopic tests familiar to any student. The presence of such abnormal constituents as blood, pus and albumen carries with it the greatest significance for the investigator.

(7) It goes without saying that much valuable knowledge about a patient's complaint may be acquired from an investigation of the cardiovascular, nervous, respiratory and alimentary systems. These systems will, of course, be examined by the practitioner in his routine examination of the patient, and need no mention here.

RADIOLOGICAL EXAMINATION

With the completion of the clinical investigation, ideally, every patient should be submitted to an X-ray examination. This, although not always possible in private practice for financial or other reasons, and not always essential in hospital, is none the less always desirable.

In many cases where calculus has not been suspected, the primary symptoms being easily explicable without the presence of a stone, one has been shown in the routine X-ray examination, thereby altering the provisional diagnosis and modifying the course of the treatment.

A complete examination of the urinary tract can often be made by a single large film of the kidneys, ureters and bladder. It will, however, usually be found advisable to have two films 12 × 10 in. in readiness, and use one for the "abdomen"

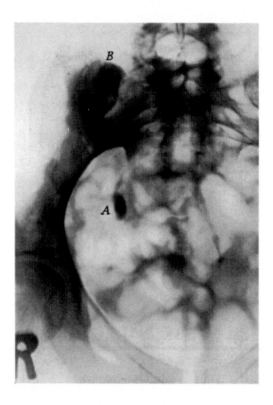

Fig. 1. X-ray showing *A*, large ureteric calculus at lower end of ureter (later passed by patient). *B*, Mass of calcareous glands.

(kidneys and ureters), and the other for the "pelvis" (bladder) and terminations of the ureters. These photographs will show most renal and vesical calculi, together with concretions in the prostate. Ureteric calculi if small and composed of uric acid may not always be opaque to the X-rays, and sometimes escape detection.

Calculi of the bladder, although often of large size, not infrequently fail to throw a satisfactory shadow on the film, which point should be borne in mind if the clinical signs indicate the presence of a calculus not confirmed by X-rays. The passage of a sound, or better still a cystoscope, should not be omitted in these cases. Considerable care and experience is necessary in the interpretation of X-ray films, and the identification of a small ureteric calculus is not always easy. Calcareous tuberculous glands in the abdomen, and phleboliths in the pelvis, are the two most fruitful sources of error in X-ray identification at the hands of a beginner (Fig. 1).

During the past ten years radiology has received most useful help from excretory urography (intravenous pyelography). This very valuable addition to urological diagnosis has been made possible by the discovery that certain iodine salts when excreted by the kidney are deposited in the calyces, pelvis and ureter, and being opaque to X-rays, throw a silhouette on the film outlining the upper "conducting" tract of the urinary system. This method consists in the intravenous injection of a solution of sodium mono-iodo-methane-sulphonate, commercially sold as Abrodil, and the taking of a series of films at short intervals after its injection. So easy of administration is this means of examination by excretory radiology that the slightly older method of retrograde pyelography has been very largely superseded, although it is still necessary for many types of cases as described in the next chapter.

Indications for Examination by Abrodil

1. To show the position of the renal pelvis, e.g. in cases of nephroptosis.

2. To show the size of the renal pelvis and calyces, e.g. in cases of hydronephrosis.

3. To show the shape of the renal pelvis and calyces in cases of renal tuberculosis, in which retrograde pyelography is undesirable. By its secretion ulcerated areas and extensions of the calyces can often be shown, particularly if a comparison with the opposite side is made. In cases of suspected growth, the encroachment of the neoplasm on the pelvis ("filling defect"), and the distortion of the calyces, can occasionally be seen. More commonly, however, retrograde pyelography will be called for owing to the somewhat poor and indefinite shadow thrown by Abrodil in these cases.

4. To show the relationship of pelvis and ureter to opaque shadows of doubtful origin, e.g. renal calculi and calcareous glands.

5. To demonstrate kinks of the ureter.

6. In cases of obscure renal infection. (Dilatation of pelvis and ureter is often present in cases of pyelonephritis.)

Intravenous pyelography rarely throws so satisfactory a silhouette as does the retrograde method. It is very valuable as a means of orientation, but is apt to fail in cases of growth, and is sometimes insufficient evidence on which to base a diagnosis of tuberculous kidney. Furthermore, where renal function is depressed, it may not be excreted at all. Conversely, the presence of a well-marked silhouette proves the presence of an actively secreting kidney. On rare occasions this method of pyelography has occasionally brought to notice the presence of a small calculus previously unsuspected. These small calculi when surrounded by Abrodil appear as small, *less* opaque areas in the denser shadow of the excreted dye.

TECHNIQUE OF INTRAVENOUS PYELOGRAPHY
WITH ABRODIL

The patient is placed recumbent on the X-ray table and all arrangements made for the taking of the photographs. 50 c.c. of Abrodil solution having been warmed to 100° F., a 50 c.c. syringe is filled with the liquid. (A tube and funnel attached to an intravenous needle will serve, although it is not so convenient.)

A superficial vein (e.g. the median basilic) having been rendered prominent by the gentle compression of a tourniquet, or better still by the partially inflated armlet of a sphygmomanometer, the needle is introduced into the vein. When blood flows from it, the solution is slowly injected—about 30–45 sec. being taken over the injection. Owing to the rapidity of excretion of the drug the injection should take place on the X-ray table, and a series of films taken 4, 8 and 12 min. after the completion of the injection. As a rule, a photograph of the abdomen after 16 min. shows a filled bladder, rendered quite opaque by the drug. Figs. 2, 3 and 4 show silhouettes of pyelograms taken from actual cases examined by this method.

It cannot be too definitely stressed that until the operator is certain that the vein has been entered, not one drop of the solution should be injected. The substance is very irritating, and if it escapes into the subcutaneous tissues a severe sloughing and ulceration will result.

The patient may mention a transient feeling of "warmth" over the whole body, occasionally progressing to a definite sweating. More rarely nausea may be complained of. Normally there are no untoward sequelae, but on the following day a mild inflammation is occasionally seen along the vein, or the skin may be reddened in the vicinity of the injection. This

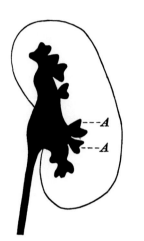

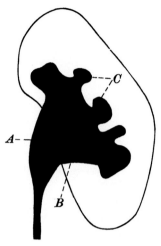

Fig. 2. Silhouette of normal renal pelvis. Note cupping of calyces, *A–A*.

Fig. 3. Silhouette of early hydronephrosis. *A*, Dilated pelvis. *B*, Wide pelviuretal angle. *C*, Club-shaped calyces.

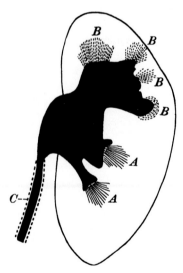

Fig. 4. Silhouette of tuberculous kidney. *A*, Normal calyces. *B*, Area of active ulceration and cavitation. *C*, Thickened and ulcerated ureter.

latter is generally due to an escape of a small amount of the drug from the vein and, though painful, generally yields to a course of fomentations and a sling.

BACTERIOLOGICAL EXAMINATION

The bacteriological investigation consists in taking a clean (catheter) specimen of urine, centrifugalizing it, and examining the deposit for bacteria and other cellular abnormalities (e.g. pus, epithelial cells and casts). Cultures can be made and growths noted.

The value of this examination is perhaps greatest when a pure growth of *B. coli communis* or *streptococcus* is found, or when tubercle bacilli can be shown to be present.

In many cases, the first specimen of urine voided through the cystoscope is drawn into a test tube, and put aside for the bacteriological examination.

BIOCHEMICAL EXAMINATION

The biochemist is called to the aid of the urologist most often when the excretory functions of the kidney are in question. The presence of a high blood urea, or low urea concentration in the urine, will draw the attention of the examiner to the impaired nitrogen-eliminating mechanism of the patient.

From the surgical point of view these biochemical tests are most likely to be invoked before operations on the urinary tract (e.g. removal of the prostate, or its resection), and a blood urea of over 50 mg. per 100 c.c. is generally considered a contraindication to a single-stage prostatectomy.

Many of these tests are in existence, and the following account from the pen of C. G. L. Wolf, Honorary Biochemist to Addenbrooke's Hospital, summarizes those in most constant use. Although they give confirmatory evidence as to the general health and renal efficiency of the patient, they are in no sense mathematically perfect, and should not weigh too heavily against an opposite opinion formed at the clinical examination.

TESTS OF RENAL EFFICIENCY IN UROLOGICAL SURGERY

To understand the reasons underlying functional tests of the kidney, it is necessary to have some idea of the physiology of this organ. Final views on the theory of secretion have not been arrived at, so that for practical purposes the practitioner can take the following description of renal tests without further enquiry as to the reasons for them.

The function of the kidney is to excrete water, which it does on an average of 1500 c.c. a day, and to a large extent controls in this way the water content of the body. Further it is employed in the elimination of certain end-products of protein metabolism. These are principally urea, uric acid, creatinine and certain compounds of unknown composition which form a considerable portion of these nitrogenous end-products.

The kidney is also concerned with the elimination of the acid products of protein metabolism, which in order to be partly neutralized are excreted combined with ammonia. It further has the duty of retaining the valuable carbohydrate, glucose, in the blood as it passes through the organ. It is evident therefore that functional renal tests may be based on the excretion of water, of urea or of some product such as creatinine or uric acid. From a practical point of view one must fix on a product whose analysis is easy of determination, and for this purpose water and urea are the two substances most commonly employed. Alternatively, one can add a foreign substance to the blood, and ascertain how much of this is excreted in a given time. The most commonly used substance of this character is phenol red, a dye of the sulphone phthalein group, which has the property, when made alkaline, of colouring the urine purple. One can by this means determine how much of a dye introduced intravenously is excreted in a given time, and from that make certain assumptions regarding the functional capacity of the kidney.

One of the earlier tests employed in assessing functional capacity was the water test used in many clinics in Germany. The method has the merit of being exceedingly simple. One has only to administer a certain volume of water under definite conditions and ascertain how much is excreted in a given time. Experience with this method shows that there are many pitfalls, and it is little used at the present moment. Estimations of creatinine and uric acid in the blood and urine have also been used, but the methods are difficult, and are only to be employed in a laboratory with skilled workers.

THE PHENOL-RED TEST

This test was introduced by the American workers, Rowntree and Geraghty,[1] in America some years ago. As has been stated above, the test is based on the assumption that the normal kidney will excrete in the first hour 40–60 per cent. of the dye injected, in the second hour 20–35 per cent., so that in 2 hours a normal kidney will excrete 60–85 per cent. of the amount of dye injected. The procedure is simple: the patient is given a glass of water about half an hour before the injection. An ampoule containing a definite quantity of the dye is opened and the contents taken up by a syringe. This is then injected either intravenously or sometimes subcutaneously. The bladder is emptied at the time of injection.

At the end of an hour the bladder is emptied, forming Test 1; at the end of a second hour the bladder is again emptied and this forms Test 2. The volumes are carefully measured. Ten c.c. of 10 per cent. sodium hydroxide are added

[1] *Archives of Internal Medicine*, 1912, vol. IX, p. 284.

to each; both solutions are then made up to a definite volume and compared with a standard solution of the dye made alkaline in a colorimeter. From the results of these two estimations one may formulate an idea regarding the functioning of the kidney. Apart from the technical difficulty of this test, the evidences of kidney failure are not brought to view so early as with the tests subsequently to be described. On the other hand, if the surgeon is waiting for signs of improvement in a case, it is possible that the phenol-red test will indicate this at an earlier stage than will the tests concerned with the excretion of urea.

UREA CONCENTRATION TEST

This test, which has been used very largely in England, is due in its present form to Hugh Maclean. It has the very great advantage that it can be carried out in the home, and the analytical procedure is such as can be done by the general practitioner, with a sufficient degree of accuracy to give useful results. The principle of the method is to administer to a patient whose bladder has been emptied 25 gm. of urea dissolved in water, and to estimate at the end of 1, 2 and 3 hours the concentration of urea in the urine excreted during this time. As will be seen, it is, in a sense, a test of the same character as the phenol-red test, employing as an indicator of efficiency a substance which can be estimated with greater ease than the dye. It has, furthermore, the physiological advantage that one is employing as an indicator the main waste product of protein metabolism. The concentration of urea in the urine is estimated by some simple ureometer, of which Gerrard's apparatus is as simple as any. The main point of difference between a normal subject and one suffering from nephritis is that the concentration of urea in the first hour's urine in a normal, healthy young man, aged 18–25, will be between 2 and

4 per cent.; in ages 25–45, within the same limits; and in hospital cases, definitely non-nephritic, the concentration will not be below 2 per cent., but the upper limit may not be so high as with patients not confined to bed. With nephritic cases the concentration of the urine is definitely below 2 per cent., and may be a third of that figure. The main difficulty with this test is the diuresis induced after the administration of urea, but Maclean says that, on the whole, there is little difficulty on this score, and one may avoid it, to a certain extent, by withholding fluid for, say, 12 hours, before the performance of the test.

UREA CONCENTRATION FACTOR

In perfectly normal, healthy subjects the concentration of urea in the blood may be taken as 25 mg., and the concentration in the urine as 2·5 per cent., so that in the excretion of urine the concentration has increased about a hundredfold. It is obvious, therefore, that one ought to be able to assess, in some measure, the function of the kidney by determining the concentration of urea in urine and blood. If this is done, and the blood urea concentration divided into the urine urea, a figure is obtained which represents to some degree the normal functioning of the kidney. This was done many years ago by Ambard, in a rather complicated way, and he claimed that one could, by his method of calculation, determine with mathematical exactness the state of the kidney at the time the test was done. The method, ingenious as it was, did not find favour either in America or in England, although undoubtedly the principle underlying the method was to a certain extent correct. A simpler method has been used in this country, largely on the suggestion of Maclean. It is the simple calculation of dividing the blood urea concentration into the urine urea concentration. Assuming that ratio

of concentration of 74 is a normal level, the cases investigated
are assessed with this figure as normal, hence a concentration
of 35 would represent a damaged kidney, and lower dividend
than this would indicate greater disturbance of function. This
method of calculation is simplicity itself, and gives on the
whole values which correspond with the clinical condition.
One must, of course, be certain that the patient is not in a
state of diuresis when the test is performed, and some of the
Canadian workers advise withholding fluid for a period of
12 hours before the test is made. One may consider this a step
in the right direction. In cases of impending prostatectomy,
the estimation of the urea in the blood alone has been largely
used. It is claimed, and with considerable justification, that
any case in which the blood urea is above 70–75 mg. per
100 c.c. is a hazardous risk. Where the bladder is being
washed out or there is considerable residual urine with
ammoniacal fermentation, the estimation of the blood urea
is the only method available.

The most satisfactory method of assessing the functional
capacity of the kidney, not only in medical but in surgical
cases, is to perform a urea clearance test.

UREA CLEARANCE TEST

This method, which has been sponsored by Donald Van Slyke[1]
and his colleagues, is in some respects a variant of the Ambard
method. Given the average normal blood flow through the
kidney, and the normal excretion of urea per minute in the
urine under definite conditions, and also knowing the urea
content of the blood, it is possible to estimate the number of
cubic centimetres of blood which would pass through the
kidney and be completely deprived of their urea content by

[1] J. P. Peters and D. D. Van Slyke, *Quantitative Clinical Chemistry*,
Baltimore, 1931, 1932.

passing through that organ. Using this as a norm the results found in nephritis can be compared with the normal figure, and it can be noted whether the total functioning tissue of the organ is active, or whether a certain portion is no longer working. The evidence Van Slyke gives for his method is convincing. By the removal of one kidney the total functional capacity drops to about 50 per cent. The method of carrying it out in clinical practice is simple. The patient needs no preliminary preparation. Urine is passed at a certain hour, and this is discarded. A sample of urine is then collected of exactly an hour's duration. A blood sample of about 5–10 c.c. is taken from the arm, and another sample of urine is collected for exactly another hour. In this way two samples are obtained which ought, in the circumstances, to be of nearly equal volume and of equal urea content. They serve as a check on one another. The blood is analysed for urea and the two samples of urine are measured for volume, and the urea content determined.

The output of urine per minute is ascertained, and with this figure, and the urea content of the urine, and of the blood, by means of a comparatively simple calculation the percentage of active, functioning tissue of the kidney can be determined. In order to avoid this calculation, Van Slyke has prepared a nomogram from which the percentage function can be read off by taking the dividend of the blood urea into the urinary urea and connecting this figure with a figure giving the outflow of urine per minute. In this nomogram anything between 120 and 80 per cent. of average normal function is given as a normal rate, below this one must consider that the kidney is functioning under less than normal conditions, and one may assume that a kidney working under less than 30 per cent. of average normal function would be a bad surgical risk.

LABORATORY METHODS FOR DETERMINING UREA IN BLOOD AND URINE

With the exception of the urea concentration test, where all that is necessary is a rough determination of the urea in the urine, the practitioner will be well advised to have the analytical procedures carried out in a laboratory, where these methods are in constant use. The rough determination of urea in the urine is made by one of the many types of apparatus of which Gerrard's modification is the most simple. The urea is decomposed with an alkaline solution of sodium hypobromite, a volume of nitrogen gas is evolved, and from this volume the concentration of urea in the urine may be easily determined, either by a table provided or by calculation. Many objections have been raised to this method, and with some reason. As the hypobromite also decomposes the ammonia of the urine its nitrogen would be added to that of the urea. Hence, in many laboratories, the ammonia is first adsorbed with permutite and the urine then submitted to the hypobromite test. The most satisfactory determination of urea in the urine, by the hypobromite method, is the recent one of Van Slyke, but as this requires a very special and expensive apparatus, the test can only be performed in a properly equipped laboratory.

The determination of urea in the blood is more difficult, and can be carried out by either of two methods. One depends upon the principle that the urea can be transformed into ammonia by means of the ferment urease which is found in high concentration in the soy or jack bean. The blood is treated under appropriate conditions with soy or jack bean for a definite time, and the ammonia so formed is removed by a current of air into a known volume of standard acid.

Part of the acid is thus neutralized, and the unneutralized portion is determined with standard alkali. A description of the method and the apparatus employed will be found in any standard text-book on biochemical methods. The method is one of very considerable accuracy, but requires some training in order to carry it out satisfactorily. Where the newer method of Van Slyke is employed, the blood proteins are precipitated and the solution from which the proteins have been removed is analysed for urea in a Van Slyke apparatus. The method is given in the *Treatise on Clinical Methods* by Peters and Van Slyke.[1]

These authors also give a full description of the urea clearance estimation, complete with nomograms to be used for calculation, and in addition a full discussion of the principles and deductions to be drawn from the performance of this test.[2]

SUMMARY

To summarize, the preliminary investigation should consist of:

1. Patient's complaint.
2. History.
3. An examination of tongue, abdomen, rectum, or vagina.
4. Examination of the urine for sugar, blood, pus, albumen and casts.
5. An X-ray examination of the urinary tract.
6. Further investigation by means of Abrodil may be carried out if the question of hydronephrosis, nephroptosis, or doubtful calculus arises; or if a tumour of doubtful nature is found and confirmatory evidence as to its renal origin is desired.
7. Renal efficiency should be tested if the rectal examination has revealed an enlarged prostate.
8. A bacteriological examination may be called for if pyuria or bacilluria are found to be present.

[1] *Loc. cit.* Methods, p. 564.
[2] *Loc. cit.* Interpretations, p. 345.

Chapter II

INVESTIGATION (*continued*)

METHODS OF ANAESTHESIA

The more specialized investigation of urological cases is carried out by means of cystoscope, urethroscope or other instrument inserted in the urethra or bladder.

Before the passage of any rigid instrument into the urethra, some type of anaesthesia is essential. It is not too much to say that instrumentation of the urethra carried out devoid of local or other anaesthesia is a survival of barbarism. "Gentleness" has been termed the best anaesthetic of the urethra, and, while there is no gainsaying its absolute necessity, it cannot be denied that the instillation of something a little more tangible than this valuable adjunct cannot fail to have a beneficial effect on the patient, both physically and mentally.

Local anaesthetization of the urethra is one of the simplest procedures to carry out successfully if the method here described is followed in detail. Too often it is ill-applied, or briefly dismissed as of no avail and a waste of time.

The most useful type of syringe is that devised by Canny Ryall. It consists of a glass barrel of 2 drachms capacity and a "squeeze bulb" attachment, and costs only 1*s.* 6*d.* This, together with a penile clamp and anaesthetizing solution, is the total armamentarium for local anaesthetization of the urethra in the male.

The solution found most useful is the following:

Cocaine hydrochloride	**gr.** vi
Sodium bicarbonate	**gr.** vi
Chloretone	**gr.** iii
Aq. dest. ad.	℥. iiss

It rapidly deteriorates and should be freshly made. One to three minims of adrenalin chloride solution may be added immediately prior to use. If the solution is made in two bottles, with the cocaine and chloretone in one and the bicarbonate of soda in the other, and mixed just before use, it will keep much longer, but not indefinitely, and the resultant mixture should always be examined before administration for precipitation, and, if this is present, discarded. Not more than 4 drachms of this solution should be used at any one examination of the patient.

No fear need be felt for the danger of cocaine poisoning. In many thousands of cases at All Saints' Hospital, London, and over two thousand cases treated elsewhere by the writer, no case of this was witnessed. It will be noted that the concentration of cocaine in the urethra is only 0·5 per cent., and the total amount of cocaine $1\frac{1}{5}$ grains. It is in amounts and concentrations greater than this that the evil effects of cocaine are to be feared.

The method of application is important. The patient having, where possible, emptied his bladder, the penis is cleansed by swabbing with 1/6000 oxycyanide of mercury solution. The syringe, containing 2 drachms of the anaesthetic, is introduced into the external urinary meatus, and the bulb gently compressed until half of this solution (1 drachm) has been slowly instilled (Fig. 5). The thumb and forefinger of the left hand, which have been holding the glans penis, then gently compress the meatal lips to prevent escape of the anaesthetic, and the syringe is temporarily laid aside.

The thumb and index finger of the right hand are now substituted for those of the left, while the left hand grasps the penis and compresses the solution into the perineum. The right hand is then freed from the glans and squeezes the fluid in the perineal urethra through the sphincter urethrae membranaceae into the posterior urethra. During this manœuvre

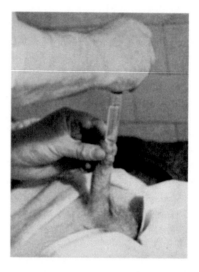

Fig. 5. Canny Ryall syringe introducing 1 drachm of anaesthetic solution into urethra extended by left thumb and forefinger.

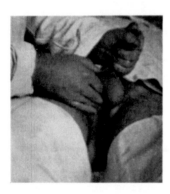

Fig. 6. Left hand grasping penis, right hand *behind* scrotum, compressing perineal urethra from before backwards.

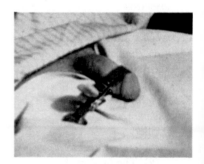

Fig. 7. Penile clamp in position to prevent leakage of anaesthetic solution from anterior urethra.

the left hand, grasping the penis in front of the scrotum, must be reached by the right hand (behind the scrotum) before compression of the contained fluid along the perineal urethra is commenced, or a pool of anaesthetic will be left between the hands in the anterior urethra and will not reach the prostate, which is the most sensitive region of the urethral lumen, and the most in need of it (Fig. 6).

The anterior urethra is now empty, and no fluid should flow from the penis if the hand is removed. This anterior urethra is then filled (at once) with the remaining drachm of fluid in the syringe, and a penile clamp applied (or if this is not available the patient can be made to compress his own meatus) to prevent the escape of anaesthetic (Fig. 7). At the expiration of 5 min. the syringe is refilled with 2 drachms, and the contained anaesthetic in the anterior urethra massaged into the posterior urethra, the full 2 drachms being then instilled into the empty anterior urethra. After a further wait of 5 min. this is massaged into the posterior urethra, and the patient is fit for instrumentation with a minimum of pain and discomfort. A successful anaesthetization should render the male urethra quite insensitive to the passage of cystoscope, urethroscope, or other metal instrument, if carried out with reasonable gentleness.

This method of local anaesthetization is highly satisfactory if carried out as described above. Too often, unfortunately, it is "modified" in one or two directions.

(1) The substitution of novocaine, or other local anaesthetic, which, although excellent when injected into the deeper tissues by means of a needle, is relatively useless when applied to a surface of mucous membrane, as it does not possess the "penetrating" power of the cocaine solution.

(2) The inefficient filling of the urethra behind the triangular ligament (urogenital diaphragm), either by allowing the solution to escape from the anterior urethra, or by inability

to conduct the contents of the anterior to the posterior urethra by efficient massage.

It must be remembered that anaesthetization of the anterior urethra is easy and rapid, but the highly sensitive verumontanum, the "trigger area" of the ejaculatory mechanism, and bladder neck, are excessively tender, and a more prolonged contact with the anaesthetic is necessary to render this region painless.

Local anaesthetization of the urethra, as described by Canny Ryall, postulates the division of the second injection (described above) into two separate drachm injections, given at an interval of 3–5 min.—making a total of three separate applications of the syringe instead of the two that the writer has found to be sufficient. Whether two or three applications are made, not more than 4 drachms are to be used, and a minimum of 12 min. (longer if desired) should be allowed between the first injection and instrumentation. Full anaesthesia lasts 10–15 min. after this.

So valuable is this local anaesthetic when properly administered, that on using it on cases of acute urinary retention caused by urethral stricture, the writer has on more than one occasion found the strictural spasm so relieved that before the catheter has been passed the patient has been able to micturate without more ado.

The female urethra, owing to its short and comparatively straight course, can be successfully anaesthetized with a pledget of wool soaked in the solution and inserted into the urethral meatus by means of a probe.

This method of anaesthesia has been found ample for the performance of observational cystoscopy, urethroscopy, urethral dilatation with bougies, sounds, and Kollmann's dilator, ureteric catheterization, and diathermy of small vesical papillomata. In some cases of tuberculosis when the bladder is contracted, non-distensible with fluid, or very sensitive, a spinal or general anaesthetic may be necessary. These cases are, however, the exception, and local anaesthesia should be employed wherever possible. Gentleness in the passage of instruments has already been referred to. In no region of the body is daintiness of touch so desirable, or so necessary, as the urethra, unless perhaps we except the eye itself.

SPINAL ANAESTHESIA

The description of spinal anaesthesia, heavy and light, would be out of place in this manual. It is, however, the anaesthetic of choice for resections of the prostate, diathermy of large papillomata, and painful operations at the bladder neck where complete anaesthesia cannot be obtained by local surface anaesthesia, for cases of litholapexy, and cystoscopy in severe degrees of cystitis (generally tuberculous).

EPIDURAL ANAESTHESIA
(Caudal block, Sacral anaesthesia)

This method (in vogue in certain special hospitals) is somewhat difficult, and not without danger in the hands of the novice: nor is it always reliable. It consists in the deposit round the spinal nerves and outside the dura mater of an anaesthetic fluid, usually 2 per cent. novocaine. The needle is entered between the sacrococcygeal hiatus, and 15–30 c.c. of a 2 per cent. solution injected. It is of the nature of a high nerve block, and should not be attempted until some previous experience has been acquired by observing and assisting at its administration by an expert. A considerable delay (15–20 min.) occurs between the time of injection and full anaesthesia.

CYSTOSCOPY

This is the examination of the inside of the bladder by means of an instrument designed for irrigation, illumination and observation. Many types of cystoscope are made, and it is obviously impossible for the practitioner to possess each modification of this highly specialized and expensive instrument. Nevertheless, the possession of a suitable observational cystoscope is well worth while to every medical man with a conscientious desire to examine his patients as thoroughly as possible.

Cystoscopes are now made in metal containers which are sterilizable by boiling, and are therefore both aseptic and ready for use in a few minutes. These cystoscopes have only recently come on the market, and as a rule one has to be content with the unboilable model which, before introduction into the urethra, must be sterilized by placing in a jar of oxycyanide of mercury (1–6000) for at least 10 min.

Cystoscopic Technique

From choice, cystoscopy is most satisfactorily carried out in the lithotomy position, the examiner standing between the knees of the patient. This can be easily managed on an ordinary operating table with lithotomy crutches, but the cystoscopic table (shown in Fig. 8) is more convenient, as the buttocks can be raised and lowered by means of a ratchet attachment, and the irrigating fluid drained into an attached tray and conducted via a waste pipe to a bucket under the table. A suitable irrigator stands to hand, and a rubber tube with a metal two-way cock connects it with the cystoscope. The cystoscope may be contained in a separate jar attached to the irrigator stand, or be kept on a separate stand.

After local anaesthetization of the urethra, the patient is draped with towels, and the cystoscope is tested to see:

(1) That the light, bulb, switch and battery are in working order.

(2) That the telescope gives a clear vision, unobscured by moist optic or other defect.

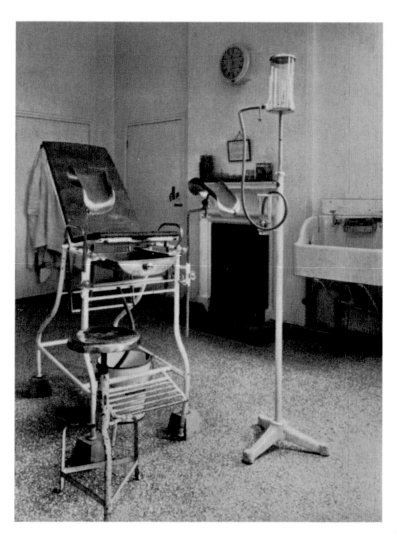

Fig. 8. Cystoscopic table and irrigator.

(3) That the collar and valve of the cystoscope are in place, and functioning.

This preliminary testing of the cystoscope before its introduction is of paramount importance. Nothing is more annoying to a patient, if not his doctor, to find after the introduction of the instrument that it has to be withdrawn to replace a defective light bulb, and re-passed a second time. The urethra is one of the most sensitive tracts of the body, and the less instrumentation it receives, the better it will behave.

The cystoscope is next lubricated: to ensure success it is necessary to use a medium which is both emollient and soluble in water. Liquid paraffin is useless for the reason that, when in contact with water, the lens is obscured and vision almost impossible. Glycerine is, in the opinion of the writer, too harsh for the delicate mucous membrane. The best form of lubricant is some compound of mucilage which is both soothing and easily soluble in watery solutions, thereby being removed from light bulb and lens when irrigation is carried out, and after it has fulfilled its function by assisting the cystoscope into the bladder. Two excellent preparations are on the market in leadfoil tubes—K.Y. jelly, made by Messrs Johnson and Johnson, and Lubafax, made by Burroughs and Welcome. A little of either, squeezed on to the beak of the cystoscope and distributed over its shank by a swab, renders the instrument slippery and well calculated to traverse the urethra with a minimum of trauma.

The operator, standing between the thighs of the patient, then lifts the penis by the left hand and inserts the beak of the cystoscope, with its contained telescope, into the meatus. Usually, it will be found best to point the beak backwards and downwards for the first inch, and then rotate the cystoscope slowly and gently through 180° so that the beak points upwards. The penis is then gently pulled on to the cystoscope, the weight of which alone should carry it down to the triangular ligament. At this point, the beak can be felt to enter the membraneous urethra, and by depressing the proximal end of the cystoscope, it can be made to traverse the prostatic urethra, and enter the bladder. No force is permissible, and though the penis may be "pulled" on to the cystoscope, this latter should never be "pushed" through the urethra.

No verbal, or written, description of this manœuvre can adequately describe it, and only by observation, and practice, can the necessary skill be acquired for a painless—and bloodless—passage of the instrument. Yet painless and bloodless it must be to be fully successful, and these two aims should be forever before the operator. When the instrument has entered the bladder, the telescope is withdrawn and irrigation begun. The two-way cock, already mentioned, is introduced through the Ringleb valve of the cystoscope and the contained urine withdrawn.

If for any reason a bacteriological examination of urine is desired, the first urine withdrawn may be run into a sterile test-tube, and the rest run into a measuring glass to note the amount of residual urine.

By moving the tap on the cock the irrigating fluid may be made to enter the bladder; about 2–3 oz. should be run in and then, by shunting the cock, evacuated into the tray (or bucket). This irrigation should be continued until the returned specimen is *absolutely clear* as shown in a glass beaker. In normal urine this may be obtained after one or two irrigations, but when pus—and even more so when blood—is present, frequent and prolonged washing may be necessary. No time is ill-spent in rendering the bladder clean, for a dirty medium is as difficult to see through as a muddy windscreen. When the medium is clear, the cock is withdrawn, the telescope reintroduced, the electric cable and switch connected, and the examination begun.

Examination. With the beak pointing upwards (as verified by the button on the proximal end of the cystoscope and telescope), the vertex of the bladder is inspected, and an air bubble—often reflecting the image of the electric bulb—seen. The mucous membrane of a normal bladder resembles the normal skin in colour, varying in tint from yellow or straw to pink, and showing marked pallor in cases of anaemia in contrast to the plethoric appearance of the robust and rubicund. The normally trabeculated appearance of the bladder roof is observed, and the presence of any abnormalities, pouches, growths or incrustations noted. Ridge pattern and trabeculation is not a prominent feature of a normal bladder but they increase with the presence of obstruction to the urinary outflow, or appear more obvious when the bladder is insufficiently filled with fluid.

By rotating the cystoscope the base is brought into view, and the two ureteric orifices on their transverse bar can be seen (Fig. 9). They should be watched until they have been in action and their efflux noted. Normally, this has the appearance of methylated spirit, or glycerine, entering water. Blood and pus descending the ureter can be easily seen. The shape of the ureteric openings should be noted, and any variations of the normal recorded. The normal ureteric orifice may vary within wide limits—"pinhole", "slit", "coffin-like" and "vulval" have been used to describe the appearance of a ureteric orifice which is in no way pathognomonic.

The widely dilated orifice of the paralysed ureter, or the trumpet-shaped opening of the retracted ureter—secondary to renal tuberculosis—can generally be recognized by the novice.

Their immediate surroundings should next be examined for oedema, injection of vessels, ulceration, and, rarely, the presence of tubercles.

Lastly the neck of the bladder and the prostate can be seen

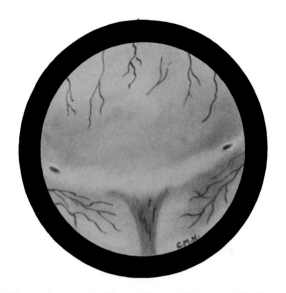

Fig. 9. Cystoscopic View of Normal Trigone of Bladder

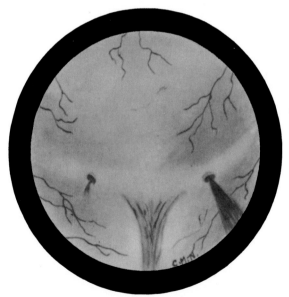

Fig. 10. Cystoscopic View of Normal Trigone showing Excretion of
Indigo-Carmine

by slightly withdrawing the cystoscope. The curtain-like projections of the prostate, though easily seen and recognized by the beginner, present pitfalls when he tries to estimate the size of the intravesical projection of this organ.

No hard and fast direction for the estimation of prostatic enlargement can be given, but the obvious knob-like encroachment of an adenoma, and the slit-like appearance of the internal meatus when narrowed by lateral lobe enlargement, together with the appearance of a collar and difficulty in viewing the ureteric orifices and vesical base, are all characteristics that the practitioner used to cystoscopy will recognize.

With the completion of the inspection, the telescope is extracted, the contained fluid evacuated, and the cystoscope withdrawn, thus completing the operation of observational cystoscopy. It must be borne in mind that even the expert sometimes meets with unexpected findings at operation— findings other than those discovered at cystoscopy. These discrepancies generally relate to size and position of a tumour, and though they naturally become fewer with experience, the facts that monocular vision alone is possible by means of the cystoscope, and that bladder size varies considerably, are the explanation of these unexpected and rather disconcerting surprises.

RENAL EFFICIENCY DYE TESTS
(Intravenous injection of indigo-carmine)

The injection of 10 c.c. of 0·4 per cent. indigo-carmine into a vein is of great value on occasions. Where the ureteric orifices are difficult to identify, the rapid excretion of this drug, by the kidneys, will make them obvious. Furthermore, as a test of comparative renal efficiency, or of the presence of a functioning kidney on one or both sides, and in the early diagnosis of renal tuberculosis, it is particularly indicated.

Glass capsules containing 10 c.c. of this drug are put on the market by Martindale, and as the fluid is already sterile, it can readily and rapidly be injected into some superficial vein during the process of a cystoscopy. As a rule, its excretion from a normal kidney and ureter begins within 3 min., but any time within 7 or 8 min. may be looked on as denoting a normally functioning kidney.

If one ureter discharges a well-marked coloration after a minute or two, and the other ureter shows no discharge, either the second kidney is absent or its function is below that of the first side. This test is obviously of great value before embarking on nephrectomy and should never be omitted, unless it is already known—and not merely suspected from some other source (e.g. previous ureteric catheterization, or Abrodil X-ray)—that the remaining kidney is present and is functioning. No definite rule can be stated as to the amount of kidney tissue capable of excretability, but a rapid and deep blue coloration presupposes an actively functioning kidney. The rhythmic discharge of this ink-like fluid from the ureteric orifice presents one of the prettiest pictures in cystoscopy (Fig. 10). If successfully injected into a vein (e.g. the median basilic), no ill-effects follow, but its deposit in the subcutaneous tissues is irritating and apt to cause sloughing. Due care is therefore needed in its administration. Its excretion is made use of in the diagnosis of several conditions which need not be stressed here, but its two most useful applications are to demonstrate the position of ureters, and to determine the presence of functioning kidneys.

CATHETERIZATION OF URETERS

Catheterization of ureters is one of the most elementary of "operative" cystoscopic procedures.

Indications. (1) To determine the nature of the bacterial content of one or both kidneys (e.g. in the early stages of renal tuberculosis). (Tubercle bacilli, having been found in the bladder urine, with few bladder signs, it may be necessary to determine which kidney is affected and if one is free from infection.)

(2) Retrograde pyelography. When, for instance, intravenous pyelography has failed or given an equivocal picture.

(3) To determine the capacity of a hydronephrosis. (Usually where the Abrodil pyelogram has been unsatisfactory.)

(4) To drain, or to apply medication to the renal pelvis or ureter. (Injection of collargol, or lubricants for calculi.)

(5) To localize a shadow in the skiagram which may be a ureteric calculus (opaque bougies being used).

The catheterizing cystoscope consists of an ordinary observation cystoscope to which has been added a channel—or two if the cystoscope is of the double catheterizing type—for the ureteric catheter. This is guarded at the proximal end by a short bent tube with a stop-cock and perforated "collar". The collar is a cap-like screw with a central perforation and a rubber washer to grip the catheter, and thus prevent **bladder** urine trickling down the *outside* of the catheter to the receiving vessel and contaminating the **ureteric** urine from *inside* the catheter.

At the distal end of the cystoscope, just proximal to the light and telescope window, is a tilting hinge activated from the proximal end by a metal disc (the Albarran lever). This metal disc possesses a small metal "button" to indicate whether the hinge is raised or flat, which should be duly noted before withdrawing the cystoscope at the end of the examination (Fig. 11).

A catheterizing cystoscope having been introduced into the bladder, and the beak rotated downwards to the trigone, the ureteric orifices are sought and a catheter introduced into the channel of the cystoscope. The ureteric catheter must be suitably sterilized before introduction, and its lumen proved to be patent by the aspiration through it of some (preferably antiseptic) fluid. One method of effecting this is to introduce the distal end of the catheter into a beaker of 1/6000 oxycyanide of mercury, and having aspirated a little of the fluid by means of a syringe, leaving the proximal end to hang over the end of the sterile table and drip into a receiver, or bucket, on the floor. If this is left for 10 min., efficient sterilization of the catheter lumen can be ensured.

The catheter, having been "fed" along the barrel, will appear in the field of vision as it emerges into the bladder.

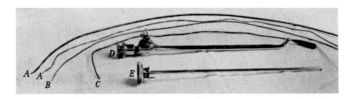

Fig. 11. Catheterizing cystoscope with ureteric catheters, opaque bougie (graduated), and diathermic electrode. *A–A*, Ureteric catheters. *B*, Opaque ureteric bougie. *C*, Diathermic electrode. *D–E*, Cystoscope.

When this is noted, the ureteric orifice is again identified and the catheter pushed straight on until it appears *beyond* and *behind* the ureteric orifice. The Albarran lever is then depressed and the point of the catheter brought up to the ureter and gently insinuated. The finger and thumb of the free hand then gently push the catheter, or bougie, up the ureter until the desired distance is reached. It will generally be found helpful to return the Albarran lever to the "flat" position after the catheter has entered the ureter, though it may need depressing from time to time—depending on the ease with which the catheter enters the ureteric lumen.

Several difficulties may be encountered—usually one of the following:

(1) One or both ureters indistinguishable by reason of inflammation, or distortion of the bladder by a much enlarged prostate or cystocele.

(2) Obstruction of ureter (e.g. pin-hole opening, stricture, kink, calculi or oedematous swelling preventing the entrance or passage of the catheter).

(3) Extreme tenderness, or apprehension on the part of the patient.

It is obvious that as experience increases the number of ureters that remain unidentified rapidly diminish, and the injection of indigo-carmine will render them obvious—unless hidden in a cystocele or behind a large prostate. A further distension of the bladder with irrigating fluid, a finger in the vagina, or a change of position, will often bring them into view when hidden at the first observation.

In the presence of some organic obstruction, a stricture of ureter or urethra may be dilated, a ureteric calculus lubricated, or the meatus slit up with scissors or electric meatatome, which latter can be introduced through the ordinary catheter channel of a catheterizing cystoscope. Extreme nervousness is best overcome by the use of a general anaesthetic. Numerous minor manœuvres designed to overcome these difficulties are commonly employed by the expert, and can be rapidly acquired by the careful student.

RETROGRADE PYELOGRAPHY

As has previously been mentioned, the intravenous injection and excretion of Abrodil has largely superseded the older and more difficult methods of retrograde (ureteric) pyelography. Nevertheless, the latter is still called for in certain cases; cases in which for some reason the excretion has been insufficient, or the silhouette too indefinite to form a just opinion of the ruling condition. Such abnormalities as "filling defects" in the renal pelvis—caused by growth or stone—usually need a retrograde pyelogram for their demonstration. Large hydro-

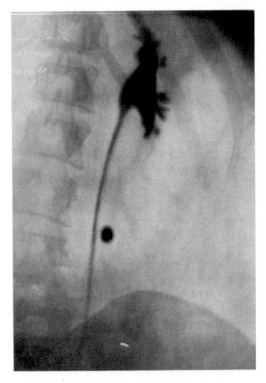

Fig. 12. Pyelogram of normal kidney showing "shadow of doubtful origin" some distance from ureter. Shadow proved to be calcareous gland.

nephroses may so dilute the excreted Abrodil that no shadow is thrown on the film, or sometimes excretion from a particular kidney may be entirely absent owing to functional inefficiency.

Ureteric conditions, e.g. kinks and obstructions, are, in general, only imperfectly demonstrated by intravenous pyelography, and may call for injection of the ureter from its vesical end.

Indications. The common indications for some type of pyelography are the following:

(1) Suspected growth of the kidney.
(2) To show the position and shape of the kidney when a palpable swelling of doubtful origin is present.
(3) To demonstrate the relation of the renal pelvis and ureter to shadows of doubtful origin in a previous skiagram (e.g. the differential diagnosis between urinary calculi and calcareous deposits in gland or vein).
(4) In cases of suspected hydronephrosis and nephroptosis.
(5) In cases of renal colic where a stone is not visible in an ordinary skiagram.
(6) Rarely, in cases of undiagnosed abdominal pain.

When for any reason in the presence of the above indications intravenous pyelography has failed, or is likely to fail, retrograde pyelography will be called for.

Contraindications. There are no absolute contraindications to intravenous pyelography, if we except extreme youth and acute general infections.

Retrograde pyelography, however, has certain definite contraindications, the following being the chief:

(1) Acute inflammation of the kidney, bladder, or urethra.
(2) Severe chronic urinary infections, particularly if associated with urethral stricture.
(3) Renal tuberculosis, when well advanced.
(4) Extreme youth.
(5) Patients who at a previous instrumentation have reacted violently, with the exhibition of rigors, high temperature, suppression, or profuse haematuria.

The main diagnostic points which may be acquired from a pyelogram are very briefly mentioned here.

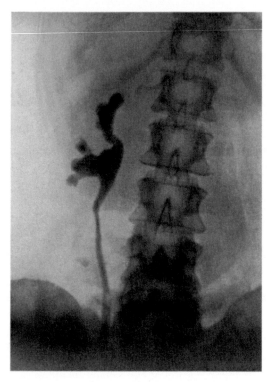

Fig. 13. Retrograde pyelogram of normal kidney.

THE NORMAL RENAL PELVIS

Thompson Walker—quoted by Roche—gives the following five guides to the study of a pyelogram (Fig. 13):

1. The normal renal pelvis is trumpet-shaped, and is vertically placed on the ureter, while the calyces project from it laterally and antero-posteriorly.

2. The normal calyx has a short neck and an expanded end, the apex of the pyramid (renal papilla) protruding into the calycal cup. While most calyces are seen projecting outwards, a calyx may be seen on end, and then appears as a round dark patch, which may simulate the shadow of a stone, near the outer margin of the pelvic shadow.

3. The opaque catheter enters the upper calyx vertically, or with a slight outward inclination.

4. The outer line of the ureter forms with the lower margin of the pelvis and lower calyx a symmetrical semicircular curve.

5. The pelvi-ureteric transition is gradual, and there is nothing to show where pelvis ends and ureter begins.

It must be borne in mind, however, that there are many variations of the normal pelvis, experience alone differentiating between the regular and the pathological.

1. **Hydronephrosis.** In advanced cases of hydronephrosis the diagnosis is obvious. The large diffuse shadow and the amount of fluid injected together with an absence of the normal calyces give a diagnostic picture which leaves nothing to the imagination. In the earlier cases, considerable experience is necessary in the interpretation of the pyelogram, the following points being worthy of notice:

(a) The terminal calycal cups become convex instead of concave, or knob-like, with thickening and shortening of the calyces.

(b) The increased amount of fluid which can be instilled into the renal pelvis without pain together with general enlargement of the pelvis.

(c) The pelvi-ureteral junction may be abrupt, and the semicircle normally found at this region may become angular (Thompson Walker's "4th guide" quoted above).

2. **Nephroptosis.** The low position of the kidney and the presence of kinks in the ureter are made manifest.

3. **Renal Growths.** In cases of a growth encroaching on the renal pelvis a "filling defect", or considerable distortion

and separation of the calyces, may be observed. The lumen of one or more of these latter may become so thin as to be almost linear in appearance, and drawn out towards the margin of the kidney. It should, however, be stressed that a retrograde pyelogram is far more likely to show these two characteristics of renal neoplasm than a skiagram taken after the injection of Abrodil (Figs. 14, 15).

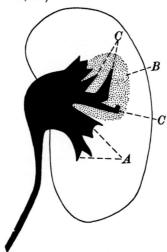

Fig. 14. Silhouette of small growth of kidney. *A, A*, Normal calyces. *B*, Area of growth. *C, C, C*, Calyces distorted by growth.

Technique

The technique of retrograde pyelography is rarely difficult. It consists in the catheterization of a ureter with the instillation into the catheter of a 14 per cent. solution of sodium iodide in water. This solution is non-irritating, non-toxic, and throws a good shadow on the X-ray plate. If preferred Abrodil half the strength of that used for intravenous pyelography may be used (i.e. 20 per cent.).

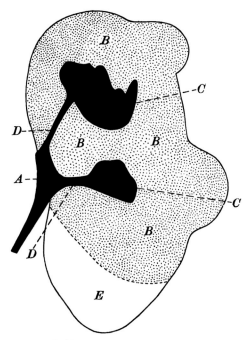

Fig. 15. Silhouette of kidney practically destroyed by very large growth. *A*, Lower pole of pelvis. *B, B, B, B,* Massive growth invading upper part of pelvis (hypernephroma). *C, C,* Necrotic cavities in growth. *D, D,* Small channels at upper and lower extremities of pelvis communicating with necrotic cavities. *E,* Normal kidney.

Before attempting this method of examination, several points should be borne in mind:

(1) General anaesthesia should never be employed.

(2) The X-ray photograph must be taken on the cystoscopic or operation table.

(3) A smaller medium-sized opaque catheter only should be used.

(4) The normal renal pelvis has a capacity of 4 to 7 c.c. Over-distension results in pain in the back.

(5) A glass syringe of 10 c.c. capacity with a terminal eyed needle is the most convenient method of injection in the hands of one skilled in cystoscopic methods. For a beginner, the fluid should be run in by gravity from a height of about 3 ft. above the patient.

(6) Injection should be stopped the moment the patient experiences the slightest pain in the back. Rupture of the pelvis from forcible over-distension has proved fatal.

(7) If no pain is experienced after the injection of 10 c.c. a pyelogram should be taken unless the kidney is known to be hydronephrotic; a further injection being carried out if no backflow down the ureter is noted and there is no complaint on the part of the patient, and a second skiagram taken when the pelvis is filled.

The patient having been prepared as for an ordinary skiagram and cystoscopy, the X-ray film is placed in position on the cystoscopic table, and the single catheterizing cystoscope is introduced. The inspection of the bladder is carried out after lavage, any abnormalities noted, and the ureteric orifices identified. A ureteric catheter is then introduced on the side of the desired pyelogram and is gently pushed up the ureter until it is arrested. This will usually be in the pelvis of the kidney, but occasionally ureteric kinks or twists may obstruct the passage of the catheter at a lower level. It is well to withdraw the catheter about 1 cm. after its arrest, as its entry into one of the calyces might give rise to considerable distortion and a misleading pyelogram result. Some authorities recommend the aspiration of the pelvic contents as they lead to dilution of the medium and a less opaque shadow results. Although there appears to be no objection to this, it is not, as a rule, necessary.

The injection of fluid into the catheter is now commenced,

preferably by an assistant, the patient being instructed to say at once if he feels any pain in the back. The cystoscopist can meanwhile observe the ureteric orifice and note the backflow of fluid (if any) which may occur round the small or medium-sized catheter used. This backflow can be taken as an indication that the pelvis is full to overflowing, even in the absence of lumbar pain, and the photographic exposure may then be made. If a graduated syringe, or burette, is used the amount run into the kidney pelvis can be noted. The injection should always be carried out very slowly and stopped when there is a complaint of pain. In hydronephroses many cubic centimetres or even ounces may be injected without any return from the ureter or any feeling of pain on the part of the patient. In such cases it is important either to leave the catheter in after the taking of the skiagram until the kidney has emptied, or better still to aspirate the contents of the large hydronephrotic sac. Where the pelvis is not markedly enlarged, retention of the catheter *in situ* for a minute is ample for the drainage of the injected fluid.

URETHROSCOPY

The examination of the urethra is carried out by means of the urethroscope. Many types of this instrument exist, but some modification of that of Geiringer (Fig. 16) is the one most commonly in use. It consists of a straight hollow tube through which is passed an introducer which acts as an obturator, and by reason of its hinge can be made to form a solid angled "beak", thereby assisting the urethroscope to enter the bladder. When this has been effected, the introducer is withdrawn and a "bundle", consisting of telescope, electric light, and irrigating channel, is introduced into the barrel. A side-cock, coupled to an irrigating flask, allows fluid to enter and distend the urethra. In most urethroscopes a hollow channel for the introduction of a diathermic electrode or ureteric catheter is also present. This, when not in use, can be occluded by a rubber cap.

The patient is placed on the cystoscopic table, as for cystoscopy, after the urethra has been anaesthetized. The urethroscope and its obturator are placed in the urethra and gently introduced until the beak can be felt to enter the posterior urethra. The outer end of the urethroscope is then depressed, and by very gentle pressure the inner end can be made to enter the bladder when no obstruction is present. The obturator is withdrawn, and telescope, light and irrigating channel introduced in its place. The irrigating fluid having

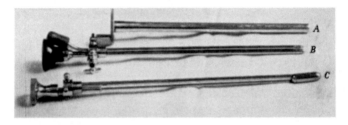

Fig. 16. Geiringer urethroscope. *A*, Barrel. *B*, "Bundle" consisting of light, lens system, irrigation channel, catheter channel. *C*, Introducer.

been connected, the side-cock turned on, and the electric cable fixed in position, observation can be commenced.

If the urethroscope is in the bladder, only a dark blur will be seen until its withdrawal to the internal urinary meatus. At this point the vesical exit can be observed and its surroundings, i.e. prostate, noted, particular attention being directed to any abnormal prominences, and to the shape of the bladder neck.

Paralysis or incompetence of the sphincter vesicae can be noted, the opening remaining round and patent—instead of the normally closed star—after the further withdrawal of the urethroscope. As the steady withdrawal continues, the prostatic urethra comes into view, and the verumontanum on the lower (posterior) wall can be identified.

From time to time it may be necessary to advance the urethroscope, and if the process is carried out under a continuous irrigation, the comfort of the patient's bladder must receive consideration in the form of frequent emptyings through the barrel of the urethroscope.

As the urethroscope is gradually and gently extracted the walls of the urethra may be examined for signs of hyperaemia, inflammation, ulceration, obstructions and false passages. In cases where a marked stricture is present and the urethroscope cannot be advanced beyond it, the face of this barrier can be inspected and the small and often elusive opening of the urethra traversing it identified.

The most common conditions which call for the use of a urethroscope are strictures, the presence of false passages, obstructions round the bladder neck, and to determine the conditions prevailing at the bladder outlet.

CYSTOSCOPY AND URETHROSCOPY IN THE CONSULTING ROOM

With the adoption of local anaesthesia and the possession of the necessary instruments, examination of the urethra and bladder can be carried out easily in the consulting room. If for any reason the cystoscopic table is not available the useful, though in the writer's opinion not ideal, substitute can be made of the ordinary examination couch and a large sandbag or stiff pillow.

The patient lies recumbent, with the buttocks well raised on the sandbag and the thighs separated. The examiner stands at the side of the patient and the cystoscope is introduced from that aspect.

The washout must of necessity take place into a receptacle between the patient's thighs, this receptacle being emptied

from time to time into a bucket conveniently placed at the
side of the couch. Some difficulty may be experienced where
the prostate is large and there is insufficient room between
the perineum and the couch in which to depress the cystoscope,
while such operations as ureteric catheterization are very
much more difficult to effect painlessly in the recumbent
than the sitting posture. Apart from these more difficult
manœuvres, the passage of a cystoscope in the consulting
room is no more difficult than the passage of a sound,
and is of infinitely more value even if an absolute and
final diagnosis cannot invariably be effected.

Chapter III

THE DIAGNOSTIC SIGNIFICANCE OF CERTAIN COMMON SYMPTOMS AND THEIR INVESTIGATION

The manifestations of urinary diseases are for the most part clear-cut and definitive, often pointing the road to diagnosis before any examination is undertaken.

The patient may approach his doctor with a complaint of one or more ills, for example frequency, pain and pyuria. Not uncommonly, however, predominance of one symptom (e.g. haematuria) may bring the sufferer to the surgeon with the single complaint of blood in the urine. In view of their great diagnostic significance, and inasmuch as each of the symptoms later to be described may have an origin in more than one organ, it has been deemed advisable to include them in a single chapter.

PAIN

Any attempt to classify pain is at best an unsatisfactory procedure, owing to its widely different appreciation on the part of sufferers; but inasmuch as three entirely different *varieties* of pain or discomfort are the usual concomitants of urinary disease, it may not be out of place to include a short section on their significance.

Pain may occur in, or be referred to any part of the urinary system. It may vary greatly both as to its cause and nature, and one exciting agent may give rise to more than one type of pain (e.g. calculus).

Type 1. A dull aching or dragging pain may be present in the loin with a kidney enlarged from any cause (e.g. hydronephrosis, pyonephrosis, tubercle, growth or large calculus).

The kidney may be tender on pressure, and is more likely to be so when the cause of its enlargement is inflammatory or due to distension of its pelvis. It is probable that the backache present in cases of renal swellings is due to the continual pull on one of the constituents of the renal pedicle—to wit, the sympathetic nerve supply which consists of a well-marked strand of fibres placed for the most part on the anterior aspect of the renal artery. The same type of chronic aching pain may be found in the perineum, associated with infections of the prostate and posterior urethra. In these cases the prostate may be found to be acutely tender on rectal examination, and the pain is due to vascular engorgement.

Type 2. Not to be confused with the above type is the excruciating pain of renal and ureteric colic. The passage, or attempted passage, down the ureter of a calculus gives rise to the most severe and distressing anguish to be found in any disease. It is due to the violent contractions of pelvis and ureter in their attempt to extrude a foreign body. It is associated with sweating and vomiting, and during the attacks a rigid abdominal wall is generally present. This, however, is not tender as in peritoneal irritation, and may be entirely absent in the intervals between the colic. The pain may radiate along the line of the ureter to the groin, thigh, scrotum and labium. This radiation to scrotum and testis was originally thought to be due to the passage of a calculus across the genito-femoral nerve where this lies behind the ureter and on the psoas muscle. In view of more recent knowledge, however, it appears likely that the pain in the testicle is reflex in character and due to sympathetic innervation from the same or nearby source as that of the kidneys.

Pain similar to this may occur in conditions sometimes referred to as Dietl's Crises, and has been attributed to the effect of a highly mobile kidney pulling on adhesions connected with pylorus or bowel, or to torsion of the kidney pedicle, or kinking of the ureter. It should, however, be mentioned that these supposed causes have a somewhat insecure foundation in fact.

Type 3. A third distinct type of pain is that often referred to on the part of the patient as cutting, scalding, or lancinating. It occurs just before, during, or after micturition, and is associated with an abraded or highly inflamed mucous membrane of the vesical trigone or urethra. Ulcers and infections in these regions are the common causes, although urine with a high acid or oxalate content may sometimes incite it. It is difficult, or impossible, to allocate all pain generated in the urinary system to one of the above types. The discomfort, if not actual pain, felt by a patient unable to empty an overfull bladder is a case in point. The difficulties of accurate classification, however, are not of great moment, and it is rather with the view to furnishing some basis of interrogation of the patient by the surgeon that the three above-mentioned types have been briefly outlined.

FREQUENCY

Frequency, alone or in conjunction with other symptoms, is the commonest complaint of patients suffering from urinary disease. By it is understood a condition in which the urine is voided more often than is usual for that particular patient; each micturition emptying the bladder of a relatively small amount of urine. It is not to be confused with the recurring "overflow" of surface water from a retained and distended bladder. It may occur during day and night, or be limited to the waking or sleeping hours. It is usually associated with pain or scalding on passing water, bacilluria, or pyuria, and may vary from the nocturnal frequency of two or three times—characteristic of the commencing prostatic enlargement—to the distressing 10–15 min. frequency of the severely ulcerated bladder in secondary tuberculosis.

It may be looked on as symptomatic of an irritable bladder base and neck, and is most frequently found in cases of prostatic enlargement, ulceration of the bladder, cystitis and urinary infections sometimes without gross pus. It should be borne in mind that its true significance, as has already been mentioned, is irritation of the vesical trigone, though this irritation may be, and usually is, secondary to some other condition situated higher up in the urinary tract.

Common Causes. Frequency is most commonly associated with the following conditions:

(1) Enlargement of the prostate in males.

(2) Bacillus coli infection of the urine (nearly always an infection descending from the kidneys).

(3) Renal tuberculosis.

(4) Vesical calculus.

(5) Haematuria.

(6) Pouches of the bladder.

(7) Cystocele in females.

(8) Neurological conditions. (Rarely.)

From this table it can be seen that the trigonal irritation, which results in the outward and visible sign of frequency, is close at hand in such conditions as vesical calculus, prostatic enlargement or cystocele; while it is more remote in the case of a vesical pouch emptying its infected contents on to the sensitive trigone, and still more distant in cases of renal infection with tubercle, coliform bacilli, or other organisms.

Investigation. Routine examination, previously described in chapters I and II, will of course suffice to clear up the causes of practically every case of frequency; but it may not be out of place to stress certain important points sometimes overlooked by the beginner, and even occasionally by the experienced:

(1) As has previously been suggested, the possible confusion of frequency with "overflow" might occur, and where any

obstruction to the urinary outflow is suspected it is well to bear in mind the possibility of a distended and overflowing bladder which may be the real cause of the patient's complaint of too frequent micturition. Every house surgeon must sometime or other have been painfully aware of the obstinate patient who refuses, or objects to, proposed catheterization on the ground that "he makes too much water".

(2) Retention and overflow having been excluded as far as possible by abdominal palpation and rectal examination, a skiagram of the urinary tract will generally exclude or prove the presence of calculi.

(3) Gross pus or blood in the water will need investigation on their own behalf, and are probably the cause of the patient's frequency when they occur. If they are not present a cystoscopy may reveal the presence of trigonal inflammation and, in many cases, e.g. enlargement of the prostate, stone, or tubercle, the primary cause of it.

(4) If, however, no obvious cause is found, a bacteriological examination of a clean specimen of urine may reveal a bacilluria on microscopy or culture.

RETENTION

Retention of urine may occur in three types:

         (a) Acute.
         (b) Chronic.
         (c) Retention and overflow.

(a) **Acute Retention** is one of the most painful and distressing conditions to which man is heir. Its commonest causes are:

(1) Urethral stricture.

(2) Enlargement of the prostate.

(3) Acute urethritis—generally gonococcal in origin.

(4) Impaction of a stone in the urethra or bladder neck.

(5) Urethral trauma, e.g. rupture or instrumentation of an irritable urethra.

(6) "Reflex" retention may occur after operations particularly in the region of anus, rectum, inguinal canal and perineum. The condition is well recognised by any dresser as a common post-operative complication which, however, rarely persists for more than a day or two.

(7) The ingestion of certain drugs (e.g. cantharides, hexamine, or potassium citrate) in susceptible individuals occasionally results in an attack of acute retention.

It is characterized by severe hypogastric pain, urgent desire to pass water and the inability to effect this.

(b) **Chronic Retention** is evidenced by increasing difficulty in passing water and the inability to empty the bladder completely, resulting in a certain residuum of urine being left behind at the end of the act of micturition. Difficulty in commencing the act, smallness or distortion of the stream, and lack of projectile power, are often referred to by the patient. Its most common causes are enlargements and irregularities of the prostate, and urethral stricture.

(c) **Retention and Overflow.** This interesting condition, although usually of grave significance, is not by any means invariably painful, and may on occasion exist without the patient suspecting it, and with comparatively little discomfort. It consists of a bladder distended with urine, which periodically voids a small amount of surface water just as an overfull bath can overflow down the waste pipe. It would appear that two types of this condition are possible:

(1) *The painful*, in which the patient probably notices a hypogastric swelling, but which he is loath to attribute to a full bladder as he is continually passing a small amount of urine—usually only a few drachms at a time. It may be associated with a rather oedematous urethra. The urine is often grossly infected, and even when instrumentation has

not been attempted a small amount of blood may be present in the urine.

(2) *The painless.* In the second type, the patient may be quite unaware of any urinary abnormality until the doctor draws his attention to a hypogastric swelling. He may be passing water regularly, in moderate amount and free from infection, but the swelling does not disappear and he is suffering from a quiescent and painless condition of retention and overflow. This condition would appear to be rather of the nature of excessive residual urine than of true retention and overflow.

From time immemorial the amount of residual urine possessed by a patient has been held to be in direct proportion to the gravity of his case, and only the most fearless, or rash operator, would consider it safe to perform a single stage prostatectomy, for example, where the residual urine measured more than 6 or 8 oz. It has been found that the burden thrown on the kidneys in these cases has so impaired their excretory capacity that the extra stress of an operation has resulted in their cessation of function with the sequela of surgical uraemia. Nor is retention and overflow confined to the male sex. In some cases this false frequency may be the first sign of a retroverted gravid uterus, and in others a cervical fibroid may so obstruct the female urethra that retention and overflow result.

Although properly the province of the gynaecologist these two conditions are not uncommon and should be borne in mind when a woman who may be pregnant or possess a fibroid complains of unduly "frequent" micturition.

All three types of retention—acute, chronic and overflow— may occur in certain lesions of the nervous system, the two commonest being tabes and disseminated sclerosis; while gross paraplegic conditions are notorious for the frequency with which they call for catheterization.

Investigation. Investigation of urinary retention carries with it certain pitfalls. The reckless passage of a catheter in an acute gonorrhoeal urethritis may result in the spread of the disease to bladder, vesiculae, or epididymis. In extremely wasted and elderly men with a large soft prostate and overflow retention, catheterization may be the surest way of effecting their demise. These untoward results should at least be considered before the casual passage of a catheter is attempted. To the careful observer the diagnosis of retention is obvious, and investigation directed towards its *cause* should be the first consideration.

Inspection and palpation of the abdomen will generally bring to light the presence of a distended, and often tender bladder. As a rule this is about half way between umbilicus and pubis before the doctor is called in, but in cases of overflow retention may be considerably larger—reaching to the umbilicus or even above it. The examiner should always attempt to define the upper limit of the bladder by the ulnar border of the hand. The perfunctory percussion of the anterior abdominal wall in front of the bladder is to be deprecated as a means of diagnosis, as it is apt to lead to errors in interpretation of the percussion note. Even skilled clinicians, depending on percussion alone, have overlooked a full bladder which should have been demonstrable by palpation. Only in the fattest of subjects is a distended bladder likely to be missed, when the possibility of the condition is borne in mind and a hypogastric tumour sought.

Where acute urinary infection is absent and gross trauma can be excluded, by far the commonest causes of retention are prostatic obstruction and post-gonorrhoeal urethral stricture. The indications and contraindications for the passage of a catheter will be described under their appropriate section, and the causal conditions alone considered here.

A history of a urethral discharge of recent date, or a long-ago

gonorrhoeal infection, will direct the attention of the surgeon
to an acute urethritis or post-gonorrhoeal stricture. A rectal
examination in the male should never be omitted: in the
female a vaginal examination will be more helpful. The
enlarged prostate, retroverted uterus and cervical fibroid can
be detected by the examining finger. A ruptured or damaged
urethra cries aloud for recognition, while in retention of
nervous origin the past history of the case and a neurological
examination make the diagnosis of the cause reasonably
certain.

A cystoscopy will most often be called for in those cases
where the obstruction is prostatic in origin without much, or
any, enlargement of this organ into the rectum. The "middle
lobe", "prostatic bar", and "collar" formations of the
prostate may be the cause of the condition, and can be
determined only by the use of the cystoscope. Where a
urethral stricture or other obstruction is present which cannot
be traversed by sound or catheter, a urethroscopy may be
helpful in bringing the face of the stricture and its elusive
opening to ocular inspection, or in demonstrating the presence
of a stone or foreign body occluding the urethra.

Skiagraphy is rarely called for in the diagnosis of these
conditions, but a calculous prostate, if not suspected by the
examining finger, will be shown on the X-ray film.

RESIDUAL URINE

Although properly not a symptom, and certainly not a
complaint on behalf of a patient, residual urine plays an
important part in the diagnosis and prognosis of certain
symptoms. It may be defined as the measure of urine which
can be drawn off by a catheter immediately after the patient
has voluntarily emptied the bladder of all that he is capable.
This residual urine will vary from a few drops in a child to
many ounces in an old man with an enlarged prostate. The

amount is in direct proportion to the gravity of the disease, indicating dilatation and failure of bladder musculature, and impairment—potential or actual—of renal function.

Its pathology is not clear, and although several theories as to its presence have been advanced, they do not appear to be founded on very sure evidence. The suggestion that residual urine is a pool lying in a post-prostatic bay of the bladder and left behind when the urinary tide falls, although picturesque, is not borne out by fact. It would perhaps be more satisfactory if we considered residual urine to be part of an essential stimulus to micturition when the threshold of bladder evacuation is raised. It is conceivable that a bladder with obstruction to its outlet acts much in the same way as the embarrassed heart, first dilating and then compensating this dilatation by hypertrophy of its walls. Such a bladder will be stimulated to empty itself only by an increased internal pressure, and it may be that when the contents of the bladder have fallen to a low ebb, the internal stimulus is no longer of sufficient intensity to continue vesical contraction. A residuum of urine is therefore left behind which will become greater as vesical dilatation outstrips its mural compensation.

As has already been suggested in a previous paragraph, excessive residual urine blends imperceptibly with the painless type of retention and overflow. Whatever the cause, its significance is great and is one of the most valuable pointers in deciding the nature of the treatment in prostatic enlargement. A residual urine of more than 4 oz. is commonly a deciding factor against one-stage prostatectomy, and though no hard and fast rule can be dictated, the beginner will do well to consider amounts greater than this of serious import. As the amount of residual urine rises, certain other physical signs (e.g. trigonal hypertrophy, and trabeculation of the bladder walls—often with the presence of small pouch-like diverticula) become manifest on cystoscopy.

INCONTINENCE

Incontinence has been divided into "true" and "false". False incontinence is identical with distension and overflow. It has already been dealt with in a previous section. True incontinence may be active or passive.

Active incontinence, sometimes referred to as the automatic bladder, and generally following late after some spinal injury, resembles the flush-tank action of a water closet—the bladder filling up without the patient's knowledge, and emptying itself at periodic intervals when the unconscious stimulus is great enough.

Passive incontinence is the slow continuous dribbling from a bladder which never fills, and is due to some interference with the bladder sphincter—organic or functional. Herein lies its significance and, in its investigation, attention should be directed to conditions which may hamper the sphincter vesicae in its normal action (e.g. organic disease of the prostate, epispadias, or interference with its nerve supply).

By urethroscopy, sphincteric paralysis can be appreciated immediately—the widely dilated and circular opening of the internal urinary meatus which fails to contract when the urethroscope is withdrawn gives a picture diagnostic of this condition. Gross irregularities in prostate or bladder may be identified by the same means, or in certain cases by cystoscopy, while the history of the case may direct attention to the nervous system.

HAEMATURIA

Haematuria is the presence in the urine of blood. An *appearance* of blood in the urine may be found in **haemoglobinuria**, but in this condition clotting is absent and no red corpuscles are found. The possibility of haemoglobinuria should be borne in mind after the ingestion of certain drugs (e.g. senna, sulphonal or rhubarb), and a microscopic examination of the urine undertaken.

True haematuria may occur from many agencies and sources, the four main causes being:

1. **Trauma to any part of the Urinary Tract** (e.g. Rupture of the kidney, or instrumentation of urethra and bladder).

2. **Stone in any part of the Urinary Tract.** (Commonly associated with pain, pus, or frequency, but calculi in the renal parenchyma may cause haematuria which may be entirely painless.)

3. **Growth—Innocent or Malignant—of Kidney, Bladder or Prostate.** (Growth of kidney rare. Papilloma and carcinoma of the bladder are the commonest causes of haematuria in man; enlargement of the prostate not uncommon.)

4. **Inflammatory Conditions of the Urinary Tract** (e.g. *B. coli*, tubercle, streptococci). (Commonest causes of haematuria in women.)

In addition to these main causes, less frequent and indefinite origins of haemorrhage may be found, for example:

(a) "Essential" renal haemorrhage (renal epistaxis).

(b) Following the ingestion of certain foods, e.g. rhubarb, gooseberries, strawberries and spinach.

In this case the haemorrhage is probably the result of a mechanical irritation by excessive amounts of oxalates.

(c) Purpura.

(d) In acute and chronic nephritis.

(e) Polycystic kidney.

(f) Varicose veins of the bladder.

Haematuria may occur alone, or may be predominant to other present symptoms. For example, painless haematuria occurring alone may be indicative of a renal or bladder growth. On the other hand, if the haematuria is associated with pain—particularly if colicky in nature—it may suggest a calculus descending the ureter. If pus and frequency are added, a vesical calculus will be a likely cause.

From this it can be seen that the examination of a patient with haematuria carries with it the determination of its site of origin, and where possible the investigation should take place at the earliest possible moment, preferably whilst bleeding still continues. Too often do we hear of the patient being fobbed off with the remark: "If the bleeding does not stop soon, we mnst have you examined by a specialist." Many cases of early growth of the bladder give rise to slight haemorrhage which rapidly ceases and perhaps does not recur for months, with the result that much valuable time is lost and the patient's life jeopardized.

Every case of haematuria where general diseases (e.g. nephritis or purpura) can be excluded, should be submitted at once to a routine examination as laid down in chapters I and II.

In view of the great importance, and prevalence of haematuria as a presenting symptom, the following rough scheme of examination, with the conclusions to be drawn from it, is appended. It must be borne in mind that the conclusions are only suggestions and taken alone are insufficient evidence on which to base a judgment.

A. *Interrogation*

  (i) Duration.

 (ii) Trauma. Rupture or bruising of urinary tract.

(iii) Pain absent. Growth of kidney, bladder or prostate.

(iv) Pain present. Stone and ulceration of bladder.

 (v) Relation of pain to haemorrhage. If pain precedes haemorrhage, probably due to stone; if following haemorrhage, to the passage of clots.

(vi) Frequency slight, or absent. Haemorrhage in upper urinary tract.

(vii) Frequency well marked. Denotes irritation, infection, or ulceration at base of bladder.

(viii) Exercise. Little or no effect except in kidney or bladder stones.

B. *Clinical Investigation*

Clinical investigation of the abdomen may reveal an enlarged or tender kidney which *may* be the site of the haematuria (e.g. in growth or infection of the kidney). It must not, however, be forgotten that an enlarged or tender kidney may result from the impaction of a calculus low down in the ureter. Still more important, when renal tuberculosis is present—especially in advanced cases—the enlarged kidney may be the healthy and hypertrophied organ doing the duty of two. Ignorance of this point has led in the past to the removal of the sound and compensated organ in mistake for the diseased kidney which may be the smaller. A rectal examination may bring to light an enlarged or calculous prostate, and advanced growths of the bladder. In the female, a vaginal examination may locate a low ureteric calculus.

C. *X-ray Examination*

Whenever possible, an X-ray examination of the urinary tract should be carried out. Renal and vesical calculi are generally well shown on the X-ray film, although small uric acid calculi in the ureter may not be opaque to the X-ray. Omission to have a skiagram taken may occasionally result in the site of the haemorrhage being allocated to some organ other than that responsible for it. Particularly is this likely to happen when the examination of the patient is carried out after the cessation of the haemorrhage, and when, for example, a moderately enlarged and soft prostate is discovered on rectal examination. It must be within the recollection of some surgeons that a case of painless hae-

maturia thought to be prostatic in origin, and submitted to
an unnecessary prostatectomy, has later been found to be due
to a calculus embedded in the renal parenchyma.

D. *Cystoscopic Examination*

The cystoscopic examination will reveal the presence of
growths of the bladder, enlargement or growth of the prostate,
injection of vessels and ulceration in the bladder wall, and
tubercles when present (rarely) round the ureteric orifices.
Varices may be noted, but they should not be accused of
being the origin of the haemorrhage unless they are actually
seen to be bleeding at the time of examination. If the
haemorrhage, though still continuing, is not proceeding from
a vesical or prostatic source, the bloody efflux from one ureter
will localize the affected kidney. It will readily be realized
that those cases of renal haematuria which come to the
surgeon after the cessation of bleeding are the most difficult to
diagnose, and it is in these particular cases that the inexperienced may rather hastily attribute the cause to the presence of
varicose veins of the bladder, or enlargement of the prostate.
No case of haematuria of suspected, but unproved, renal
origin should be discharged until a pyelogram has been taken.

E. *Bacteriological Examination*

The first specimen withdrawn from the cystoscope can, if
necessary, be submitted to the bacteriologist, and a hitherto
unsuspected bacilluria may be found to account for the
haemorrhage. The writer is strongly of opinion that the
proper time for the bacteriological examination is during, and
not before, cystoscopy. It may be a great temptation on the
part of a keen pathologist to withdraw a catheter specimen
of urine from a case of haematuria and submit it to bacteriological examination, and on finding it to be infected with
B. coli, for example, to have a vaccine prepared and the

patient inoculated—thereby possibly overlooking a stone or papilloma of the bladder.

PYURIA AND BACILLURIA

Pus may occur in the urine from an infection in any part of the urinary tract, or by rupture into it of an abscess situated outside it. The term bacilluria implies the presence of bacteria in the urine without gross pus. The commonest causes of pyuria are:

(1) Infections of the kidney and its pelvis, usually associated with stone, or ureteric obstruction, and pyonephrosis.

(2) Infection of the bladder, either secondary to a descending renal focus or associated with stone, pouch, or enlargement of the prostate.

(3) Infections of the urethra and prostate—generally gonococcal in nature—give rise to a discharge of pus which will appear in the urine, and in the case of a urethritis may escape from the urinary meatus independent of micturition.

Intermittent pyuria may occur in conditions of pyonephrosis and vesical pouch when periodic discharges of pus may be liberated. The investigation of pyuria is similar to that previously described for haematuria, but a word of warning should be uttered against the passage of a cystoscope in the case of a gonococcal urethritis with the consequent spread of infection that will result.

PNEUMATURIA

Pneumaturia is the passage of gas at the end of micturition. It is much more frequent in men than in women. By far the commonest cause of this condition is the development of an intestino-vesical fistula—generally malignant in origin, although less commonly resulting from inflammatory conditions of the colon such as diverticulitis.

Very rarely a single discharge of gas may occur after

instrumentation of the bladder with the consequent introduction of air. Still more rarely, it may occur from the
fermentation of sugary urine by certain bacteria, e.g. *B. coli
communis* or *B. proteus*. In many cases it is associated with
a severe cystitis from the passage of faecal matter in the urine.

When due to an intestino-vesical fistula, cystoscopy will
usually reveal a swollen and oedematous area of the bladder
which surrounds the fistulous opening into the bowel. Unless
faeces are in process of being extruded from it, the opening
itself is generally obscured by the surrounding oedema.
A barium enema and sigmoidoscopy may, on occasion, render
valuable information as to the site and nature of the bowel
involvement. When—on rare occasions—the condition is due
to urinary fermentation, a test for sugar will reveal this fact.

HYPOGASTRIC TUMOUR

The presence of a cystic swelling above the pubis is mentioned
here only to remind the student of the two commonest causes
of this condition—the distended bladder, and the pregnant
uterus. The importance of an overfull bladder, sometimes
unsuspected until a catheter has been passed, has already
been stressed.

Differential diagnosis is from such conditions as "fibroids"
of the uterus, ovarian cysts, pelvic abscess (generally resulting
from perforations of appendix or bowel) and, rarely, hydatid
disease in this region.

A careful attention to the history of the complaint with a
rectal or vaginal examination, together with the passage of
a catheter, will suffice to render the diagnosis clear. It is well
to bear in mind that a combination of conditions may
occasionally occur; for example, an early retroverted gravid
uterus with a distended bladder, or a uterine fibroid situated
in the cervix by compression on the female urethra, may give
rise to retention and overflow.

Chapter IV

THE KIDNEY

ANATOMY

The kidneys are retroperitoneal organs situated in the loins, and placed in front of the last two ribs and the diaphragm, psoas and quadratus lumborum muscles. That on the left side lies at a higher level than that on the right.

The pleura descends below the last rib and may be exposed posterior to the kidney in operations on the kidney from behind.

In front the kidneys are in relation with the peritoneal sac and its contents—colon and small intestine. In addition, the right kidney has the second part of the duodenum traversing its medial half, whilst spleen, stomach and pancreas lie in front of the upper half of the left. Each kidney may be looked on as consisting of a parenchymatous (or secreting portion), and a pelvis (or conducting part).

Nipple-shaped prominences of the kidney medulla (the pyramids) project into extensions (calyces) of the funnel-shaped pelvis. The total capacity of the normal pelvis without the production of pain is about 5–7 c.c.

Three capsules invest the kidney:
1. The capsule proper—thin and membraneous.
2. An investment of fat.
3. A fascial envelope passing above, in front, and behind the kidneys, and blending with the transversalis and iliac fasciae.

Blood Supply. Normally the kidney receives a single artery at the level of the second lumbar vertebra which enters the hilum of the organ between vein and ureter. Not uncommonly, however, one or more additional vessels may be present, and when passing to the lower pole behind the ureter may give rise to obstruction to the urinary outflow with consequent hydronephrosis.

The vein on the left side is three times the length of that on the right. It is crossed near its entry into the inferior vena cava by the superior mesenteric artery which arises from the aorta immediately above it.

This point should be borne in mind in cases of albuminuria in children without apparent cause and localized to the left side. The trapping of the vein between the arterial pincers (aorta and superior mesenteric artery) may partially obstruct the venous outflow, thereby damaging the secretory epithelium of the kidney.

Nerve Supply. The kidney receives its innervation (sympathetic) along its vascular pedicle—the main strands running on the anterior surface of the artery between that vessel and the renal vein, where they may be sought and severed in cases requiring sympathectomy. The fibres are derived from the lower thoracic and upper lumbar segments.

Lymph derived from the kidney passes to the lateral aortic glands.

A renal swelling presents certain characteristics. If large it can be felt and compressed between the two hands—one placed in the loin and the other on the anterior abdominal wall. It bulges towards the flank, and if mobile can be reduced into the loin. It moves on respiration, although not very freely, and a band of resonance to percussion is nearly always demonstrable across its anterior surface, due to the presence of the colon. The percussion note lateral and posterior to this is dull.

The differential diagnosis of a renal swelling is generally from spleen, or neoplasm of the descending colon on the left side, whilst, to the right of the midline, liver and gall-bladder swellings are most frequently liable to confusion with it.

URINE

Urinary secretion may vary in amount or composition in diseases which may have no connection with urological conditions. An excess of urine (polyuria) may occur continuously as in interstitial nephritis and early tuberculosis of the kidney, or intermittently in highly nervous individuals.

ANURIA

Anuria (suppression of urine) is the condition found when, for one cause or another, the kidneys cease to secrete urine, or the measure drops to such small proportions as to amount to practical suppression. The site of its origin may be:

(a) Pre-renal (e.g. hysteria, and circulatory failure from shock or other cause).

(b) Renal (e.g. after unilateral nephrectomy when the remaining kidney is found to be functionless or absent, and in kidneys damaged by infection or fibrotic change).

(c) Post-renal (e.g. bilateral impaction of calculi, or pathological changes in bladder, prostate, or urethra).

Its chief causes, however, are:

(i) Infective (a) blood borne,
           (b) ascending.
(ii) "Back pressure" (c) increase,
                    (d) decrease.
(iii) Reflex.

(i) Infections of the kidney borne to it through the blood stream (e.g. in septicaemia, scarlatina, influenza, pneumonia or typhoid) may all cause suppression of the urine, which may be serious or fatal. An acute ascending infection of the kidneys, secondary to an infective focus somewhat lower in the urinary tract, can cause fatal suppression of the urine.

(ii) Back pressure. The sudden increase in back pressure on the kidneys, for example by the simultaneous impaction of calculi in both ureters (rare), or by the impaction of a single calculus in the ureter of a healthy kidney, with an absent or severely damaged kidney on the opposite side, may give rise to urinary suppression. The gradual increase in back pressure from prostatic or strictural obstruction to the bladder outflow may eventually result in anuria. Conversely, the sudden relief of tension from the rapid emptying of an over-distended bladder by catheter—or more rarely by a suprapubic cystotomy—may be followed by a diminution or suppression of urinary secretion.

(iii) "Reflex" anuria may result from disease or trauma in any part of the urinary apparatus (e.g. the passage of sounds through a stricture, or operation on bladder, ureter or kidney). When a calculus impacts in the ureter of an otherwise healthy kidney, it may give rise to mechanical suppression of urine from the calculous kidney, and reflex suppression of secretion from the kidney of the opposite side. This second kidney, in these cases, is invariably the seat of disease—generally well advanced.

The significance of anuria is twofold: Firstly, it must not be confused with retention, and the first steps in its investigation must be to the exclusion of this contingency by examination and, if necessary, catheterization of the bladder. Secondly, the recognition of anuria carries with it the urgent necessity for the removal of its cause where this is possible.

Treatment. In circulatory anuria, raising of the blood pressure and the administration of diuretics (e.g. by copious draughts of water, gin, caffeine or salyrgan) are usually sufficient to recommence renal secretion. Pituitrin may be useful, and saline infusions into rectum or vein will be called for if oral administration of fluids is insufficient.

In infective anuria, if the above measures have failed, nephrostomy or renal decapsulation may be needed.

Where anuria results from the impaction of calculi, these must be removed. When bilateral calculi are impacted in the ureters, the side in which pain most recently occurred should be dealt with first, or simple nephrostomy established.

If anuria has supervened as the result of a too-sudden "decompression" of the kidney, benefit may result from measures taken to raise the intravesical pressure in conjunction with the general medical treatment previously mentioned. Means to this end may be effected by injecting the bladder with fluid, raising the foot-end of the bed on blocks, placing a spigot in catheter—or suprapubic tube if that is present—and withdrawing small amounts of the bladder contents at hourly intervals. As prevention of this condition is usually possible, the too-sudden emptying of an overfilled bladder is to be avoided.

In urgent cases of anuria, hot packs and injections of pilocarpine, together with intravenous saline infusions to which glucose may be added, should be tried.

URAEMIA

Uraemia is a condition which results from the retention in the blood of toxins normally voided in the urine. It may occur after surgical interference in diseases other than those of the urinary system, but its most acute manifestations are found in cases of urinary suppression or greatly diminished secretion.

At the present moment no single known substance in the blood has been found to account for the signs and symptoms referred to as uraemia. It is, however, closely connected with the presence in the blood of a high nitrogen content. It is found in its commonest form in cases of enlarged prostate, with resultant damage to the kidneys from back pressure. The patient may show a yellowish appearance, with a raised pulse, a dry, cracked, or brown tongue, and a foul breath. Hiccup may occur. The blood urea is much raised, and the urea concentration poor. In the more severe cases, intense headache and vomiting may occur. It is well to bear in mind that the vomiting may be so profuse as to resemble that of acute intestinal obstruction. Fibrillary twitchings of the muscles and convulsions are not uncommon. Drowsiness, passing into coma, is the usual termination.

Some urological cases, although not showing signs of uraemia, may yet develop these after operation. Such signs as dry and brown tongue, hiccup, thirst, headache and vomiting are not uncommon. They are generally held to be uraemic in origin and, although as a rule yielding to treatment, must be looked on as forebodings of some gravity.

Treatment. The treatment of uraemia is generally bound up with that of a greatly diminished urinary secretion, or suppression. Every effort to remove the cause of these conditions must be made. Where obstruction to bladder outflow occurs this must be remedied.

Fluid intake must be forced—preferably by mouth, failing which rectal and colonic salines must be instituted. At least 3 quarts of water should be ingested during the 24 hours, and the usual diuretics may be given.

Nephrostomy may be called for if infection of the kidneys is present, or where a previous cystotomy has failed to relieve the symptoms.

CONGENITAL MALFORMATIONS

Complete absence of a kidney is fortunately rare, but its occurrence must be borne in mind before the performance of a nephrectomy. An enlarged and compensated kidney is usually present on the opposite side, while imperfect descent of the testis may occur on the side from which the kidney is absent.

Additional kidneys are practically unknown, but lobulation with the presence of additional ureters is not uncommon.

According to Morris "horseshoe" (fused) kidney occurs once in every 1000 bodies. It is usually associated with a lowly position in the abdomen, and more than two ureters may be present.

Additional vessels are not uncommon, and calculous disease is more prone to occur in a "horseshoe", than in a normal-shaped kidney.

The diagnosis is made by palpation and radiology after the excretion of Abrodil, or the performance of a retrograde pyelogram.

Treatment is rarely called for unless concomitant disease (stone, hydronephrosis, tubercle) occurs.

MOVABLE KIDNEY

The causes of an unduly mobile kidney have not yet been fully determined. It is almost entirely confined to the female sex, and cases fall into three main groups:

(1) Those without symptoms.
(2) Those associated with general visceroptosis occurring in (a) fat, (b) lean individuals.
(3) Those with urinary symptoms: (a) renal (hydro-nephrotic); (b) vesical (frequency, scalding, pyuria).

Class 1 represents those cases in which a routine examination has brought to light the presence of a movable and prolapsed kidney, usually on one side only, of which the patient is unaware. She has no symptoms referable to the urinary tract, and if she can be left without knowledge of this condition the result is all to the good. At any rate surgical treatment should not be attempted.

Class 2 contains a large number of cases with complaint

of backache, loin pain, and general abdominal discomfort. Here the dropped kidney is part of a general subsidence, and surgical treatment, though sometimes justifiable, is generally inadvisable or meets with very little success. This group can be subdivided according to the general appearance of the individual into the fat and the lean. It is well to leave fat subjects severely alone as far as the treatment of their kidney is concerned. Probably because they are fat and the muscular and ligamentous structures friable, the chances of a successful anchorage are small, and a recurrence of mobility is likely, if nothing worse supervenes.

In the second group of this class, the lean patients, one generally finds women with a protuberant abdomen, a constricted lower chest, and a waist that would have been a credit to a previous generation. The kidney is palpable, mobile, and often at examination it is tender, palpation giving the patient a feeling of nausea. As a rule the patients are nervous, with a low threshold for pain, and a pyelogram or an X-ray examination with Abrodil shows a kinked ureter and a low kidney, the kinking of the ureter being unassociated with hydronephrosis.

Treatment of this class of patient is a difficult problem, and the institution of abdominal exercises or the support of a belt should be essayed. If this treatment should not avail the patient, some surgeons advocate a nephropexy; others a renal sympathectomy which at least has the merit of abolishing pain generated in the kidney.

In **Class 3** we have the true surgical mobile kidneys, and associated or not with other conditions have at least urological signs and symptoms, which can and should be corrected. The complaints vary, being any or all of the following: backache, loin pain, renal colic, renal swelling, frequency and pain on passing urine, and occasional haematuria. Intermittent fever may be present. These signs and symptoms owe their inception to an obstructed ureter, with or without microbic infection, and the obstruction and infection can be rectified by appropriate measures.

An aberrant renal artery passing to the lower pole of the kidney behind the ureter may cause an acute kinking and obstruction of this organ when the kidney slips downwards, with the result that a painful commencing hydronephrosis is instigated. In these cases the aberrant renal artery should be severed if it is thought (after previous temporary compression of the artery) that too great an area of the kidney will not be rendered anaemic. At any rate a nephropexy will in all probability prevent further damage to the kidney by obliterating the ureteric kink.

In other cases obstruction, kinking and fixation of the ureter may be effected by membrane-like adhesions, comparable with Jackson's membrane, and Lane's kink in the right iliac fossa. In these cases the back pressure on the renal pelvis is insufficient or too variable to produce a hydronephrosis, and the symptoms, frequency, scalding and haematuria, are the result of renal infection imperfectly drained, with secondary infection at the bladder base. Fixation of the kidney, freeing of the ureter from adhesions, followed by the administration of urinary antiseptics and, if necessary, pyelolavage by means of cystoscope and ureteric catheter, will usually effect a cure.

It cannot be too strongly emphasized that the treatment of a mobile kidney is the rectification of its obstructed outflow when that occurs. The presence of a movable and dropped kidney, *per se*, is no more harmful than a dropped "h".

HYDRONEPHROSIS

Hydronephrosis consists in a dilatation of the renal pelvis, calyces, and later cavitation of the kidney tissue itself. It may be present at birth, unilateral or bilateral, and is the result of an intermittent or partial obstruction to urinary outflow.

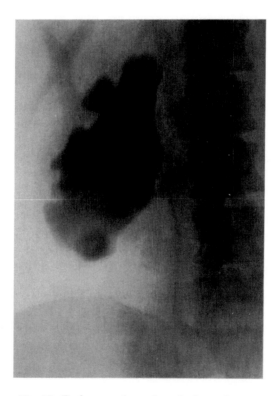

Fig. 17. Pyelogram of very large hydronephrosis
(16 oz. capacity).

The hydronephrosis may be "intermittent", "open" (when urine escapes from the ureter), or "closed" (when no urine escapes).

Causes. A sudden total obstruction of the ureter will not give rise to hydronephrosis, but rather to urinary suppression and renal atrophy. Partial obstruction, however, from enlargement of the prostate, or urethral stricture, are occasional causes of hydronephrosis—not uncommonly bilateral. Somewhat more often a vesical growth obstructing the lower end of the ureter is the cause: but the commonest of all causes are conditions affecting the upper urinary tract; for example, renal and ureteric calculi acting as ball valves, ureteric kinks from adhesions or aberrant vessels associated with undue mobility of the kidney, or stricture of the ureter from congenital or traumatic origin. Occasionally an unnaturally high implantation of the ureter into the renal pelvis is found.

Rarely, no obvious obstruction is discovered, and spasm of the ureter or pelvi-ureteral junction due to an overaction of the sympathetic system has been blamed as the cause.

Pathology. The renal pelvis and calyces which normally carry 5–8 c.c. of fluid without the presence of pain become dilated enormously, and many ounces of fluid can be injected by means of a ureteric catheter without the production of discomfort.

The pyramids, which normally project into the calyces, become flattened or hollowed out, so that a pyelogram shows the normal calycal "cups" replaced by convex or knob-like extremities, with shortening and thickening of the calyces themselves.

The renal parenchyma is greatly thinned, and may be stretched as an attenuated layer over the large cystic pelvis.

If the urinary obstruction is high up, the pelvi-ureteral junction will be well marked. If situated low down, dilatation of the ureter will be present, masking this junction.

An aberrant renal vessel passing to the lower pole of the kidney will only cause ureteric obstruction if it enters the kidney behind the ureter.

Certain types of hydronephrosis show a constricted or highly placed pelvi-ureteral junction with a hydronephrotic sac extending down far below its outlet.

Adhesions fixing a kinked ureter may sometimes be found, but rarely give rise to any but the smallest degree of pelvic dilatation.

Signs and Symptoms. Although hydronephrosis may occasionally be present without signs or symptoms, the usual case presents any or all of the following signs:

(1) An enlarged renal swelling—as a rule not tender— unassociated with a rise in temperature, and may give a cystic feel to the examining hand.

(2) Intermittent attacks of polyuria may occur, associated with lessening in size of the swelling if the obstruction is capable of being overcome from time to time.

(3) Pain is not a prominent feature, but a dull ache is sometimes complained of, and occasionally in the intermittent or more mobile type colic-like attacks may occur. There is no change in the urinary composition as a rule.

Investigation and Diagnosis. A renal, or suspected renal swelling should be submitted to X-ray. Calculi may be seen, and if impacted at the renal outlet may be the cause of the condition.

A skiagram after the excretion of Abrodil may make the condition clear, and give some indication of the function of the opposite kidney.

More commonly, a retrograde pyelogram will be necessary, when the ureteric orifice can be inspected, its condition noted, and the characteristic appearances of the hydronephrotic silhouette seen (Figs. 3, 17).

The diagnosis is from such renal conditions as:

(1) Pyonephrosis (pus and rise of temperature present);

(2) Renal growth (haematuria and character of pyelogram);

(3) Polycystic kidney (often bilateral, nodular, and character of pyelogram);
and such extrarenal conditions as liver, gall-bladder, and
splenic enlargements.

Treatment. Where the hydronephrosis is consequent on
obstruction of the urethra by the prostate or stricture—
particularly if bilateral—these primary conditions alone should
be dealt with. Similarly growths of the bladder, if present,
will need removal.

In cases where hydronephrosis has resulted from ureteric
kinking over an aberrant vessel, there is some difference of
opinion as to the type of treatment to be adopted. Division
of this artery in many cases results in the atrophy of the lower
pole of the kidney, which fact must be borne in mind when
deciding on the mode of treatment.

If a moderate amount of kidney tissue remains, and it is
thought that a nephropexy can permanently obliterate the
ureteric kink, it is obviously unwise to sever the vessel. On
the other hand, it is rare that a nephropexy alone can overcome the ureteric obstruction, in which case the artery should
be divided—some indication of the viability of the renal
tissues supplied by this vessel being gained from observing the
degree of anaemia resulting from its temporary compression.

Such obvious causes as renal and ureteric calculi should
be removed, but some more direct treatment of the hydronephrosis itself may be necessary, e.g. dilatation of the
stricture resulting from their presence.

Occasionally plastic operations on pelvis and ureter are
advisable, and possible (e.g. uretero-pelvic anastomosis, or
excision of that part of the pelvis below the insertion of the
ureter).

In many cases, however, the size of the hydronephrosis, or
the uselessness of the small amount of the remaining kidney
tissue makes nephrectomy the only possible treatment.

To sum up, the preliminary investigation will have made clear:

(1) The condition of the opposite kidney; and

(2) The likelihood of saving the hydronephrotic one.

If at operation, after the removal of any obvious obstruction (stone, kink or adhesion), the contents of the hydronephrotic sac can be emptied into the bladder by steady compression without difficulty and a moderate amount of kidney tissue remains, the organ is worth saving and can be fixed in position by a nephropexy.

If the hydronephrosis is not easily emptied of its contents by compression, or if it is very large and the amount of kidney tissue insignificant, the organ should be removed.

In certain cases of painful kidney a small hydronephrosis devoid of mechanical cause is present. These cases have been submitted to renal sympathectomy by some surgeons. It has been found that this operation undoubtedly relieves pain, and is thought to remove a spasmodic obstruction of the ureter which may be due to over-action of the sympathetic system. Be that as it may, experimental filling of a renal pelvis by ureteric catheter after denervation can be carried out to a far greater extent, without pain, than before operation: and some doubt must exist in the mind of the surgeon as to whether he has but substituted a painless hydronephrosis for some obscure painful condition of the kidney unattended by marked pelvic dilatation.

Before resorting to sympathectomy it is well to attempt the fluoroscopic examination of the renal pelvis after its injection with some substance opaque to the X-rays. In suitable cases its contractile rhythm can be watched on the X-ray screen and, after the injection of eserine, a rapid and painless emptying of its contents can be seen. (Where organic obstruction is present the injection of eserine is associated with an increase in renal pain.)

It appears advisable, at any rate before embarking on surgical treatment in these cases, to watch the therapeutic effect of repeated injections of eserine. If pain is relieved but returns when the injections are discontinued, sympathectomy may justifiably be undertaken.

RUPTURE OF THE KIDNEY

Rupture of the kidney may take place subcutaneously, or through an external wound: the former is much the more common. A history of an accident is obtained and the patient complains of pain in the region of the kidney, which may radiate along the ureter to the testicle.

Haemorrhage in the tissues of the loin may be present or may not occur for some days. The kidney is tender and a large tumour may be palpable on examination. The muscles of the abdominal wall are rigid, and signs of internal haemorrhage may be marked.

Haematuria is present in 90 per cent. of cases. Shock is variable but generally well marked.

If the peritoneum is torn, which not uncommonly happens in children, signs of peritoneal involvement are superimposed.

In cases where the opposite kidney is the site of disease, reflex anuria may occur.

Treatment. Where haemorrhage is not profuse, complete rest, tight bandaging of the side, and the administration of haemostatic serum and morphine will suffice. The oral administration of urinary antiseptics is advisable.

Where an external wound exists, excision of this and, if necessary, exploration of the kidney should be undertaken. If haemorrhage is severe, or the peritoneal cavity opened, exploration with probable nephrectomy may be necessary.

In cases where operation is not immediately called for, attention must be paid to the pulse and temperature charts, and a strict look-out kept for signs of internal haemorrhage, urinary extravasation, or the later formation of a perinephric abscess.

INFECTIONS OF THE KIDNEY

Bacterial infections of the urinary tract are for the most part blood-borne. Infection is brought to the kidney in the blood stream, from which focus it may descend in the urine or via the periureteric plexus to the lower urinary organs—bladder, prostate and urethra.

In the past it has been customary to refer to infection of a single part of the urinary tract as if it occurred alone, e.g. pyelitis. It is now more generally realized that such conditions as pyelitis in which the pelvis receives the greatest stress of infection, pyelonephritis in which the infection spreads to the kidney, and pyonephrosis in which obstruction to the pelvis results in dilatation and infection of the kidney and pelvis, are only different degrees of the same process (Figs. 18, 19, 20). Nor is there any doubt that the urinary tract as a whole suffers when its upper reaches become the seat of infective processes. This would account for the presence of such bladder symptoms as frequency and painful micturition in the early stages of pyelitis.

Furthermore, although infection of the kidney and pelvis may sometimes result from an ascent from a primary focus in the lower urinary tract (e.g. "surgical kidney"), such is not the commonest method of infection of the kidneys. Nor does an ascending infection travel up the ureteric lumen, but rather via the periureteric plexus of the lymphatic vessels.

Some observers even deny the possibility of ascending infection, maintaining that it is invariably blood-borne from a lower urinary focus. At all events renal infection is nearly always associated with some degree of obstruction to urinary outflow.

Bearing in mind the extensive nature of infections of the

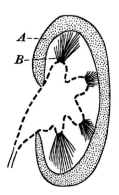

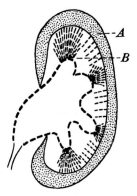

Fig. 18. Pyelitis. Main stress of infection on pelvis and calyces (shown by broken line). [Pyramids, medulla, and cortex unaffected.] *A*, Cortex. *B*, Medulla.

Fig. 19. Pyelonephritis. Main stress of infection on pelvis, calyces, and medulla of kidney (shown by broken lines). [Cortex unaffected.] *A*, Cortex. *B*, Medulla.

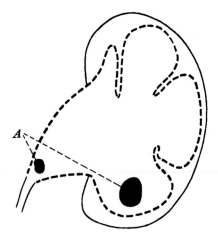

Fig. 20. Pyonephrosis. Destruction of pelvis, calyces, medulla, extending to renal cortex (with enlargement of organ). Calculi present (*A*).

kidney, the names in use are not particularly accurate descriptions of the existing condition.

The mildest type of renal infection is a bacilluria where infection of the renal pelvis with mild inflammation of the bladder mucous membrane occurs.

When pyuria is present, ulceration of the renal pelvis to a greater or less extent exists, and the occurrence of rigors, high temperature, casts and albumen (except in small amounts) will denote extension to the renal parenchyma. Tenderness of the kidney may be present without enlargement, but any marked increase in the size of the organ will denote a commencing pyonephrosis.

Notwithstanding the above remarks, for the sake of convenience these different degrees of renal infection have been described under their old headings—pyelitis, pyelonephritis and pyonephrosis.

PYELITIS

Infection of the renal pelvis and its calyces is characterized by hyperaemia of its internal lining, and by the presence of small ulcers in the more severe cases. Pus and sometimes blood is present, and some predisposing obstructive cause, e.g. calculus, growth or pregnancy can often be found. Other cases follow bouts of constipation, while it is not uncommon on the honeymoon following what Kidd has described as the "rites of the marriage bed".

Clinically mild and severe cases occur. In the milder cases, apart from frequency and painful micturition, there are few symptoms, although the kidney may be tender and the temperature raised. The signs in these cases denote a prominence on the part of the secondary (bladder) over the primary (kidney) signs.

In the severe cases frequency and pain are more intense. Haematuria may be present, and pyuria marked. Tenderness of the kidney, high temperature, shiverings or rigors become manifest, and the patient very ill. The bladder urine is generally neutral or alkaline, but if a specimen is taken by ureteric catheter from the infected kidney it is acid in reaction. Cystoscopy is rarely called for in the acute conditions, but an inflamed ureteric orifice can be seen from which a cloudy efflux of urine issues.

In the subacute and chronic stages, pain in the region of the kidney diminishes, the temperature drops, and rigors cease. Inflammation of the bladder may become more diffuse and ulceration may occur.

Pyelitis is not uncommon in infancy, and its possibility should be borne in mind when a child under two years shows pyrexia, rigors and extreme distress without other symptoms.

Pyelitis of pregnancy is common, almost invariably on the right side, and has been attributed to pressure of the foetal head or gravid uterus on the ureter. In view of the fact that pyelitis occurs most commonly during the first half of pregnancy, the suggested cause of foetal pressure would not seem entirely convincing.

Diagnosis. Cases of pyelitis are not infrequently confounded with appendicitis. The presence of a tender kidney, higher temperature, and pus in the urine, should render the diagnosis certain in most cases. It is in those cases where the symptoms are milder and pyuria less obvious in which confusion occurs.

Acute inflammation of tube and ovary may occasionally be confused with pyelitis until a urinary examination has been carried out.

Treatment. This consists in the removal, where possible, of any predisposing cause, e.g. calculus, ureteric or urethral obstruction. Rest in bed and copious draughts of barley water or cherry-stalk tea, with the administration of large doses of potassium citrate ($\frac{1}{2}$ to 1 dr. t.d.s.) is advisable in the early stages. If potassium citrate is not easily tolerated, sodium or potassium acetate may be tried. Later urinary antiseptics may be given—perhaps the most useful being hexylresorcinol, or the institution of a ketogenic diet may be worthy of a trial, although as a rule it is not well borne.

Attention should be directed to the removal of constipation, and charcoal or other intestinal antiseptic may be useful in those cases in which infection has originated in the bowel.

If a chronic and stationary condition is reached, lavage of the renal pelvis with a 5 per cent. solution of collargol introduced through a ureteric catheter is often helpful in clearing up the residual infection.

Drainage of the renal pelvis by an indwelling ureteric catheter for 48–96 hours has given excellent results in the hands of some observers, particularly in those cases where some degree of ureteric obstruction exists—including the pyelitis of pregnancy.

Pyelonephritis

In this condition there is infection both of the pelvis and the kidney parenchyma. Small abscesses scattered through the kidney rapidly make their appearance, and intense inflammation of medulla and pelvis is seen. It may occur in an organ afflicted with calculous or other disease, but not uncommonly results as an ascending infection from the lower urinary tract—often following on instrumentation or operation.

Clinically it is a more advanced, and correspondingly more serious condition than that of pyelitis. Temperature is higher, and rigors more severe. Renal efficiency is low, and the urine in addition to blood, pus and albumen generally contains casts. Suppression may take place. The kidney is tender and sometimes palpable, though palpability generally indicates commencing pyonephrosis.

After an acute attack the condition may become chronic, although liable to exacerbations from time to time.

The severity of the prognosis is directly in proportion to the amount of kidney damage sustained. Where multiple abscesses have occurred, resulting damage to the kidney tissue is severe, and some degree of chronic nephritis will remain as a permanent legacy.

Treatment. Treatment as a whole is not very satisfactory. Where the condition has resulted from an ascending infection, treatment of the lower urinary tract is generally called for and occasionally yields brilliant results. This treatment will usually take the form of bladder washes, or suprapubic drainage of the bladder.

In unilateral haematogenous cases where calculi are present in the kidney, these should be removed as soon as the patient is in a fit condition to stand the operation. The kidney should be drained by a tube placed in the pelvis. Nephrectomy may become necessary later.

In bilateral cases where general medical treatment (which is the same as that for anuria and uraemia) has failed to effect an improvement, and the patient's life is threatened, nephrostomy on one or both sides may be called for.

In the more chronic cases drainage of the renal pelvis by the indwelling ureteric catheter combined with daily pyelo-lavage is sometimes helpful. The ureteric catheter can be left *in situ* from 5 to 10 days if due attention is taken to see that its lumen is not blocked by pus or clot.

PYONEPHROSIS

When in addition to severe renal infection is added urinary obstruction, the condition of pyonephrosis occurs, and the pelvis and calyces become dilated often to a marked extent. The kidney tissue is destroyed and resembles a hollow sac full of pus in which calculi are not uncommonly found. These latter may be either the cause of the obstruction, or may be generated in the stagnant pus as a result.

The condition may be unilateral or bilateral, and may also occur as the result of pyogenic infection of a previous hydronephrosis. The ureter becomes thickened, and inflammation may extend outside the kidney with the formation of dense adhesions to the surrounding structures. Occasionally perirenal suppuration takes place.

Clinically, pyonephrosis is invariably an advance on some antecedent condition, for when after previous infection (pyelonephritis) a tender loin gives place to a tender and palpable renal swelling, or a previous hydronephrosis shows evidence of suppuration, pyonephrosis will have occurred.

Subacute and acute cases occur, high temperatures and rigors being present in the more severe cases. Pus is present in the urine, although it is sometimes intermittent in its appearance.

Investigation. Cystoscopy, which is essential, will reveal the side of the lesion and, at the same time, give some indication of the competence of the other kidney if the intravenous injection of indigo-carmine be carried out. The orifice of the infected ureter is round and immobile, and from it pus escapes. Even in cases where the condition appears unilateral, the function of the second kidney may be much depressed and its secretion poor.

An X-ray may reveal the presence of calculi, and a bacteriological examination is often of assistance.

Treatment. In unilateral cases with a competent second kidney, nephrectomy should be performed. If the patient is very ill, or the function of the second kidney defective, nephrostomy of the damaged organ with the removal of any calculi present is the operation of choice. It is unlikely, however, that the wound will heal, and the secondary nephrectomy when the patient is in a better condition to withstand further operative interference will usually be necessary.

Very large pyonephroses can often be rendered much smaller and more suitable for removal by a previous drainage.

In bilateral cases any obvious cause of urinary obstruction (e.g. stricture, or enlarged prostate) will need attention, and each case must be considered on its own merits as to whether further operation is advisable and, if so, whether unilateral or bilateral nephrostomy is to be advocated. It must be borne in mind that renal damage is severe, and uraemia sooner or later may supervene.

PERIRENAL SUPPURATION
(Perinephric abscess)

Abscesses occurring round the kidney are not very common. Three types are generally described:

1. Embolic. The infection is brought via the blood or lymphatic stream from some distant focus. A carbuncle is perhaps the commonest cause, and perirenal suppuration has an unfortunate habit of occurring as a complication in cases of epidemic influenza.

2. As a direct extension from infection of some neighbouring organ (e.g. appendix, gall-bladder, duodenum or pleura).

The above two types are sometimes referred to as "primary", since the kidney itself is perfectly healthy.

3. As a spread of infection from the kidney (e.g. from pyonephrosis, or consequent on a previous rupture and infection of the organ).

This type is often referred to as "secondary".

Dense adhesions, or the presence of fibrolipomatous masses, are sometimes found round a damaged kidney, representing the tissue reaction to a subacute or chronic infection.

Signs and Symptoms. Pain and tenderness in the loin, intermittent temperature and rigidity of the muscles of the loin, should raise the suspicion of perirenal suppuration. Swelling is present in the later stages, which may become reddened and oedematous. The hip may be held flexed and full extension may be difficult. The urine as a rule is not affected except in the secondary types.

Diagnosis. In the early stages typhoid and paratyphoid fever must be excluded, whilst in the later stages disease of the hip joint may cause confusion.

Treatment. Incision and evacuation of the pus should be undertaken as soon as the diagnosis is made. In the secondary types, where a pyonephrosis is present, drainage of the kidney should be performed at the same time. A secondary nephrectomy will usually be called for at a later date. Disease of appendix, gall-bladder, duodenum or pleura may need attention in other cases.

TUBERCULOSIS OF THE KIDNEY

See chapter IX on Genito-urinary Tuberculosis.

NEPHRITIS AND ALBUMINURIA

These conditions are generally looked on as medical diseases, but surgical urology has been helpful in dealing with two types of albuminuria:

(1) In certain asthenic children albuminuria may be found devoid of other symptoms. The children are usually poorly nourished, narrow chested, with a protuberant abdomen and faulty stance. Constipation is often marked, and the left kidney is occasionally palpable. Lordosis may be present.

On investigation by means of the catheterizing cystoscope no changes are seen in the bladder, but a specimen of urine taken from the left ureter may be shown to possess albumen, while that of the right is free from it. The albuminuria may be intermittent in type, and is associated with a trapping of the left renal vein between the aorta and superior mesenteric artery. This is brought about by the overloaded and dropped bowels dragging on the mesentery and its contained artery.

Treatment consists in regulating the bowels, overcoming faulty positions of stance, and giving massage and exercises to the abdominal and spinal muscles, together with general muscular tonics.

(2) In certain cases of chronic nephritis, and more rarely in the acute conditions, where uraemia is threatening, decapsulation of the kidney or nephrostomy may be called for. Nephrostomy is most likely to succeed where some degree of ureteric obstruction is present. Decapsulation allows the formation of anastomoses between the kidney substance and the surrounding tissues by which means a partial bypass round the kidney is produced. A consequent lessening of its engorgement, which, together with the decompressing effect resulting from the removal of its capsule, relieves some pressure from the swollen and damaged tubules, allowing them a better chance of recovering their function. Good results have been reported—temporarily at any rate.

CALCULUS

Renal calculus is a common condition, and a variety of chemically different stones may be manufactured in the kidney: uric acid, urates of ammonium, sodium, potassium and calcium oxalate are perhaps the commonest, although phosphatic stones are not unknown.

The precise chemical composition and appearance of the stone is of little moment, but calcium oxalate calculi are generally dark, knobbly in appearance and opaque to the X-rays: uric acid and urate calculi are smooth, reddish or yellow in colour and are not so opaque to the X-rays; phosphatic calculi are whitish, opaque to X-rays and are more likely to occur in the bladder than in the kidney.

Renal calculi may occur in the renal parenchyma, in the renal pelvis, or in a single calyx in which they may become encysted. A "branching" calculus, resembling a cast of the renal pelvis and calyces, is fairly common, and may exist without any symptoms drawing attention to its presence.

Causes. The causes of calculus formation in the kidneys are but imperfectly understood. The older theories of a lithiasis due to an excessive oxalate or urate intake in the dietary are no longer tenable.

Recently McCarrison, after numerous experiments, has concluded that urinary calculus is a deficiency disease due to the absence or diminution of vitamin A of animal origin in conjunction with other factors, and he has summarized his conclusions thus:

The formation of urinary calculi is dependent on the following factors:

(1) Deficiency of vitamin A derived from animal sources.

(2) Deficiency of phosphates relative to the amount of calcium in the diet.

(3) Excess of calcium.

(4) The presence of some unknown agent in whole cereal grains.

To these may be added other predisposing causes as urinary stagnation and infection: the site of this latter is not uncommonly in prostate, bladder neck, or cervix, or it may be situated outside the urinary tract.

Signs and Symptoms. Signs and symptoms of a calculus in the kidney will depend on:

(1) The position of the stone.

(2) Its mobility.

(3) The presence of infection.

A small stone embedded in the parenchyma of the kidney,

or large branching calculus filling up the cavity of the pelvis and calyces, may give no signs at all. More commonly these large calculi give rise to a renal aching, or some degree of discomfort in the loin.

A calculus situated in the parenchyma may give rise to haematuria which is often entirely painless, pain only becoming marked when the calculus begins to move. Calculi situated in the pelvis nearly always give rise to some pain, generally commencing below the last rib and travelling along the line of the ureter to groin or scrotum, often made worse by exercise or jolting. Intense colic is associated with an attempt on the part of the kidney to extrude these calculi into the ureter. (Renal colic, see p. 48.)

Infection in some degree and at some time is invariably present. It is probably both a cause and a result of calculi and may progress through the stages of renal infection—pyelitis, pyelonephritis and pyonephrosis: in which latter condition an enlarged, tender and palpable kidney will be present.

Investigation and Diagnosis. Renal calculi are not uncommonly bilateral. An X-ray (of the whole urinary tract) will, in nearly all cases, reliably demonstrate the presence of stones in the kidney. The shadows of calcareous glands and foreign bodies must be carefully differentiated from those of calculi. If haematuria or pyuria is present, cystoscopy will show from which side it is proceeding, and an indigo-carmine test will make clear the degree of functional competence of the opposite kidney.

Treatment. (1) *Prophylaxis.* The removal of septic foci —particularly if situated in the genito-urinary tract (cervix, prostate or bladder)—is always to be recommended. The presence in the diet of an adequate supply of milk, cream and butter, together with a lessening of the calcium salts, or the addition of phosphates, are points worthy of attention, particularly in cases in which gravel has occurred.

(2) *Surgical.* Renal calculi should be removed unless contraindicated, as their presence sooner or later damages the kidney by the production of a chronic interstitial nephritis with consequent deterioration of its functional capacity. Small calculi situated in the parenchyma are unsuitable for removal, and calculi in elderly patients, devoid of signs or symptoms, can generally be left.

Previous to operation large amounts of fluid should be given; cherry-stalk tea and lemonade are particularly valuable. Urinary antiseptics should always be administered, for although they have not a very marked effect on infection in the kidney, they may considerably diminish, or prevent from supervening, an infection of the lower urinary organs. Hexylresorcinol, acriflavine, neotropine and hexamine are perhaps the most favoured.

Wherever possible the calculus should be removed via the renal pelvis rather than through the posterior border of the kidney, as the so-called bloodless line of Hertyl has a habit of proving anything but bloodless when tested on the operating table.

Where multiple calculi, associated with considerable renal destruction, are present, or a large calculus has greatly damaged the kidney, a primary nephrectomy will be called for, if the function of the other kidney is satisfactory. When bilateral calculi are present the least-damaged kidney should be operated on first, and every attempt made to preserve both kidneys. It is inadvisable to operate on both sides at the same session.

When severe anuria is present as a result of bilateral calculi, or impacted calculus in a single functioning kidney, any attempt to remove the stone may prove too great a strain for the patient. In these cases nephrostomy should be undertaken at the earliest possible moment, and removal of the stone or stones deferred until the patient is in a better condition to withstand the much more serious operation of their removal.

During an attack of renal colic an operation, unless it be lubrication of the ureter, should not be undertaken. Morphia and atropine may be given, and hot-water bottles or fomentations applied to the painful side. Fluids should be encouraged unless vomiting is marked, in which case rectal salines are often helpful.

GROWTHS OF THE KIDNEY

Growths of the kidney may occur in the renal parenchyma, or the renal pelvis.

Pathologically they have been classified as innocent or malignant, but inasmuch as the innocent growths are extremely rare, do not give rise to symptoms, and are only discovered at operation or post mortem, they are of little interest to the surgeon.

The pathology of renal growths has not yet been fully worked out, and a uniformity in nomenclature has unfortunately not yet been attained. The commonest growths giving rise to symptoms are sarcoma, carcinoma, and hypernephroma, affecting the renal parenchyma, and the so-called papilloma of the renal pelvis. This is generally described as innocent, though its tendency to recurrence, extrarenal invasion and secondary implants renders it, if not of a gross malignancy, at least on the borders thereof.

Angioma of the renal pelvis is a rare condition and, though not strictly speaking a "growth", is worthy of mention as a rare cause of symptomless haematuria.

Sarcoma of the kidney may occur in infants, in whom it is not uncommon during the first three years of life. By some it is regarded as a mixed tumour of the nature of a teratoma. It may attain large proportions and haematuria is absent or slight in amount.

Sarcoma and carcinoma of adults are both rare, the latter generally being an adeno-carcinoma.

Hypernephroma, which is nowadays generally held to be a carcinoma of the renal tubules, is the commonest tumour of the renal parenchyma. It is most frequently situated at the upper part of the kidney, and consists of a nodular growth, hard in parts, but by degeneration becomes soft and cystic in others. It is usually yellow or orange in appearance and haemorrhages may occur into it. Metastases affecting the bones and lungs are not uncommon.

The villous tumour of the renal pelvis (papilloma) resembles that seen in the bladder. The base is, however, rather more intimately blended with the surrounding kidney tissue, and the villi stunted, both of which points indicate a tendency to malignancy which may not be present in a bladder growth. Secondary implants down the ureter occur, and invasion beyond the confines of the kidney is not uncommon. True metastases, however, are not found.

Signs and Symptoms. Haematuria is the first symptom in 70 per cent. of cases. It is generally painless in the early stages, although it may be associated with renal aching or ureteric colic (from the passage of clots) in the later stages. It is, however, uncommon in the sarcoma of infants and, when present, is small in amount. Renal tumour becomes manifest sooner or later, while invasion of the renal vein not only gives rise to metastases, but not uncommonly causes a varicocele to develop on that side.

Investigation and Diagnosis. Painless haematuria with the presence of a renal swelling, where stone and infections can be excluded, is diagnostic of a growth of the kidney. Congenital cystic kidney may cause confusion, but this is generally bilateral. Investigation by means of a pyelogram may be helpful, and if the growth has encroached on the cavity of the renal pelvis a filling defect or distortion of the calyces will be seen (Figs. 14, 15). This latter may take the form of "fragmentation", or a narrow irregular channel, which has been likened to the form of a spider's leg.

Treatment. Nephrectomy, if secondary growths are not present and the function of the other kidney is satisfactory.

CYSTS OF THE KIDNEY

Solitary cysts are occasionally found in the kidney, as also are dermoid and hydatid cysts. When discovered they should, if possible, be removed.

POLYCYSTIC KIDNEY
(Congenital cystic kidney)

This condition consists of numerous cysts springing from the kidney tissue, which by their growth compress and destroy the parenchyma until uraemia supervenes. The condition is generally, though not invariably, bilateral, and one kidney is often considerably larger than the other. It rarely becomes manifest before the age of forty. Haematuria is not an uncommon symptom, and a dragging or aching pain in the loin is generally present during some stage of the disease.

The diagnosis is difficult and may be impossible, but in well-marked cases bilateral renal tumour, nodular to the touch, should suggest the condition.

Pyelography may help in the investigation of these cases. The typical picture bears signs of resemblance both to hydronephrosis and growth, in that the pelvis is enlarged and the calyces distorted. These appearances, however, are usually bilateral, and the association of a bilateral renal swelling of nodular consistence and haematuria often suffices to make the diagnosis reasonably certain.

Treatment. Treatment is, on the whole, unsatisfactory, owing to the usual bilateral distribution of the disease. A nephrectomy, however, should be carried out when severe unilateral haematuria occurs, in order to save the patient's life, and if the second kidney is not palpable the disease *may* be unilateral.

ESSENTIAL RENAL HAEMORRHAGE
(Renal epistaxis)

This is a condition in which painless, and otherwise symptom-less haematuria occurs. It is unilateral and no adequate cause for it has been discovered. Only those cases of unilateral renal bleeding which, after the fullest investigation and operative exploration, reveal no cause for the bleeding should be allocated to this class. It is a common experience of surgeons that after surgical exploration of the kidney for this condition the bleeding often ceases without further treatment.

Chapter V

OPERATIONS ON THE KIDNEYS

EXPOSURE

The kidney may be exposed either through the loin, through the peritoneum, or by a combination of both methods. Wherever possible the lumbar route is used.

Lumbar Route. The patient is placed in the lateral position over a large sandbag, in order to make prominent the kidney and loin to be operated on. The under-knee and hip are flexed, and the patient maintained in position by heavy and well-filled sandbags placed under the point of the uppermost shoulder and the pelvis.

A variety of incisions for the exposure of the kidney have been described—only one of which will be mentioned here.

A vertical incision crossing the last rib at the outer border of the erector spinae descends to within an inch of the iliac crest, from which point it curves outwards and forwards parallel to this structure.

The latissimus dorsi and serratus posticus inferior are divided, and the external oblique muscle of the abdomen split along the line of its fibres. The posterior fibres of the internal oblique may need division, as will the lumbo-dorsal fascia which, to all intents and purposes, represents the posterior aponeurotic origin of the transversalis muscle.

In well-developed patients the outer fibres of the quadratus lumborum may need severing, although as a rule this muscle can be retracted inwards.

The external arcuate ligament (lateral lumbo-costal arch) passing from the last rib to the transverse process of the first lumbar vertebra may need dividing, and care is necessary to avoid opening the downward prolongation of pleura in this region.

In very large tumours of the kidney the last rib will need resection, and here again the pleura is in danger of being wounded.

The perinephric tissues are then incised well to the back of the kidney in order to avoid opening the peritoneum or damaging the colon, after which the kidney can be delivered into the wound by gentle traction assisted by compression of the anterior abdominal wall by the assistant.

Abdominal Approach. This method is not often used except for very large tumours, when the peritoneum is not infrequently pushed so far over towards the opposite side that its opening is not called for.

When, however, the peritoneal sac has to be traversed, it is advisable after opening it to make the incision in its posterior wall to the outer side of the colon, which can then be displaced medially without fear of damage to its blood supply. Infection of the kidney will contraindicate this method of approach.

After the exposure of the kidney the following operations on it may be performed:

(1) Nephrostomy.
(2) Nephropexy.
(3) Nephrectomy.
(4) Plastic operations on renal pelvis, and ureter.
(5) Nephrolithotomy.
(6) Pyelolithotomy.

NEPHROSTOMY

Nephrostomy may be called for:

(1) To drain an infected kidney or pelvis.
(2) To relieve stress on the renal parenchyma in cases of anuria and uraemia (generally associated with obstruction to urinary outflow).

When the kidney is dilated the operation may prove very simple, but in a comparatively small and fixed kidney its performance may be of extreme difficulty, and doubt may arise in the mind of the surgeon as to whether or not the drainage tube has reached its destination in the pelvis (particularly if after a day or so the urinary efflux diminishes or fails entirely).

Cabot's method is to be recommended: a malleable probe (of gallstone or uterine type), previously bent to form a **V**, is introduced through a small opening in the renal pelvis, and pushed back through the renal parenchyma until its presence can be felt deep to the cortex. A small incision is made on to this and the bulbous end of the probe extruded. A stout ligature is attached, and the probe made to retrace its course until the ligature lies in the track. The proximal end of the ligature is stitched through a large catheter (preferably winged in pattern) and the catheter pulled by the ligature until its distal end can be felt to lie in the renal pelvis. The whole operation can be carried out without displacing the kidney from its bed. Bleeding from the kidney is negligible if the catheter is of larger calibre than the aperture made for the probe.

NEPHROPEXY

Nephropexy is called for in the following conditions:

(1) Where undue mobility of the kidney is resulting in a hydronephrosis owing to ureteric angulation.

(2) Where undue mobility of the kidney is associated with a chronic pyelitis which resists treatment owing to periodic ureteral obstruction.

(3) Where undue mobility is associated with periodic attacks of pain. (Dietl's Crises.)

The kidney having been exposed from the loin, the pelvis and ureter are gently freed as low down as possible from any bands or adhesions. A strip of capsule, one to three-quarters of an inch in breadth, is then dissected from the postero-lateral aspect of the kidney from the upper towards the lower pole. This strip is left attached to the lower third of the organ. Remains of the attached capsule in the upper half of the kidney are then rolled down to form a "collar" about its middle. The posterior strip is next passed over the last rib— previously freed of its fascial connections—and the kidney pushed upwards until any kinks of the ureter are straightened out.

The strip of capsule is brought down and sutured to the capsule on the lower half of the kidney and the capsular "collar" formed on its anterior and marginal aspects. By this manœuvre the lower pole of the kidney is pulled outwards, so that the now straightened ureter will drain the renal pelvis from its lowermost point.

By denuding the upper half of the kidney, adhesions between this organ and the surrounding structures are encouraged. The opening in the loin is closed, and the patient kept on the back for three weeks at least.

NEPHRECTOMY
(Lumbar)

The kidney, having been exposed, is gently delivered into the wound and the ureter sought for as it passes downwards on the psoas muscle. This is divided between ligatures, and the ends touched with pure carbolic acid.

The kidney pedicle is then gently defined, the arteries and veins being separately ligatured when this is possible. In most cases it is advisable to leave two ligatures on the divided vessels. Curved clamps can be applied to the vessels as they enter the hilum of the kidney, between which clamps and the ligatures the vessels can be divided, the kidney freed and the wound closed.

Except in cases where infection has spread outside the kidney, or urine has been spilt, drainage is unnecessary.

It is worthy of mention that nephrectomy may be a very difficult operation where adhesions are present, and where infection—as in pyonephrosis—has resulted in great friability of the renal vessels.

NEPHRECTOMY
(Abdominal)

This may be called for when the space between the iliac crest and the thorax appears insufficient for the removal of a greatly enlarged kidney which is uninfected. The kidney having been exposed by incising the peritoneum lateral to the colon—which together with its blood supply and coils of intestine is pushed across to the opposite side—the vessels and ureter are ligated, divided and the kidney freed. Drainage, when necessary, is carried out through a stab wound in the loin. The opening in the peritoneum is closed, intestines replaced and the abdomen sutured.

PLASTIC OPERATIONS ON RENAL PELVIS AND URETER

In a few cases of hydronephrosis excision of a dependent portion of the pelvis below the ureteric orifice may be called for, or an anastomosis carried out between this part of the sac and the upper part of the ureter. The method generally adopted resembles that of gastro-duodenostomy. Other cases where ureteric stricture is a marked feature may be benefited by incising the stricture, with suture along a line at right angles to the incision to increase the ureteral calibre.

For details of the technique of the several plastic operations on pelvis and ureter the reader is referred to works on operative surgery.

NEPHROLITHOTOMY AND PYELOLITHOTOMY

These operations consist in the removal of a calculus from the kidney substance (nephrolithotomy) or from the renal pelvis (pyelolithotomy). Wherever possible pyelolithotomy should be undertaken, as shock and haemorrhage are reduced to a minimum and, as the kidney is not damaged, a consequent fibrosis will not result.

Stones unsuitable for this method of removal are those which are embedded wholly—or to a large extent—in the renal parenchyma, in which case the kidney must be split along a plane just posterior to its meridian (bloodless line of Hyrtl) in the lower half of its convex border. Even with an assistant compressing the vascular pedicle of the kidney this incision is often anything but bloodless.

The kidney having been exposed and freed as far as possible from adhesions and fascial connections, it is brought into the wound and palpated. If the stone cannot be felt the kidney may be needled and the characteristic grating will demonstrate its position.

If pyelolithotomy is decided upon, the pelvis is isolated by gauze packs and an incision made on to the stone, which is gently withdrawn. The incision in the pelvis is closed with an intestinal needle when the surgeon has satisfied himself that no other calculi remain, and a tag of fat is sewn over the closed incision. The kidney is returned to its bed, and the wound in the loin closed in layers. A drainage tube down to the kidney is advisable for 48 hours.

When nephrolithotomy is necessary, or if palpation and needling have failed to reveal a calculus, the kidney may be opened as previously described and the calculus sought and removed. Suture of the kidney is carried out by thick catgut stitches passed through the substance of the organ and tied about the postero-lateral border. A drain tube down to the kidney is inserted and the wound closed. Particular watch should be kept for the appearance of undue haemorrhage after the patient has returned to bed.

Chapter VI

THE URETER

ANATOMY

The ureter commences at the lower point of the renal pelvis and passes down the posterior abdominal wall, lying in front of the psoas muscle and genito-femoral nerve. It lies behind the testicular or ovarian vessels and other vessels running to the right or left colon.

The ureter is adherent to the posterior surface of the peritoneum and remains attached to it when that membrane is displaced. It crosses the bifurcation of the common iliac artery and enters the pelvis in front of the sacro-iliac joint. At the level of the ischial spine it turns forwards and inwards, passing beside the lateral fornices of the vagina. In the female it is crossed above by the uterine artery, in the male by the vas deferens. After running obliquely through the wall of the bladder for about three-quarters of an inch it terminates in the ureteric orifice at either extremity of Mercier's bar.

Nerve Supply. The ureter receives its nerve supply from its lower end, and any periureteric plexus that may be found higher up has ascended from its lower extremity. Its innervation is similar to that of the bladder—sympathetic (lumbar II and III) via the presacral nerve, and parasympathetic (sacral II, III and IV) via the pelvic nerves.

The normal ureter is about the size of a quill pen in diameter, and is impalpable on clinical examination.

Pathologically it may become thickened or dilated until it reaches dimensions comparable with those of the intestine, in which case it may be palpable on the posterior wall of the abdomen, or in the lateral vaginal fornices.

URETEROCELE

This condition, really a prolapse of the mucous membrane of the ureteral wall, has the appearance of a cyst-like swelling in the position of the lower extremity of the ureter, varying in size from a pea to that of a walnut. A small nipple-like projection on the cyst indicates the ureteric opening which is invariably much contracted. The condition results from stenosis of the ureteric orifice. Calculi are occasionally found in its cavity.

Symptoms are irregular, and usually consist of frequency, pain in the kidney of the same side, with occasional attacks of haematuria.

Treatment consists in incising the cyst by diathermy or cystoscopic knife. Dilatation of the ureter should follow.

INJURIES

Injuries to the ureter may occur subcutaneously (e.g. crushing or stretching) but are rare. The commonest type of ureteral injury results from accidental damage during surgical operations on the pelvic organs (e.g. uterus and vagina), but wounds of the ureter have been recorded following a forceps delivery.

Symptoms and Investigation. In subcutaneous injuries pain and tenderness in the loin or along the course of the ureter are present. Urine is extravasated and a swelling may be discovered. Operation should take place at once and the ureter repaired if possible.

A preliminary cystoscopic catheterization will materially assist in localizing the lower segment of the ureter when complete division has taken place. The wound should be drained. If from sepsis or other reason a persistent ureteric fistula remains, nephrectomy will be necessary at a later date.

In surgical damage a urinary fistula sooner or later makes its appearance either through the laparotomy scar or into the vagina. If there is doubt as to the urinary nature of the fistula, the oral administration of methylene blue with the resultant coloration in the discharge will render the matter clear.

The appearance of the ureteric orifice at cystoscopy and the insertion of a catheter into the ureter will help in localizing the side and the distance from the bladder at which damage to the ureter has taken place.

The intravenous injection of indigo-carmine may be of value both in demonstrating the absence of urinary efflux on the damaged side, and the presence of a functionally capable kidney on the opposite side.

If there is reason to suppose that a partial damage to the ureter is present (as evidenced by a small outflow of urine from the fistula), it is advisable to pass a ureteric catheter, which may be left *in situ* for 5 or 6 days, and to await the result.

If the ureter is completely severed it is generally impossible to unite the severed ends unless this be attempted at the time of the severance.

If much sepsis is present the kidney of that side will sooner or later become infected, so that the methods of dealing with this condition generally resolve themselves either into a ureteral transplantation into the sigmoid, or a nephrectomy after previously ascertaining the functional capacity of the opposite kidney.

ADHESIONS

Adhesions about the ureter usually take the form of a vascular membrane, similar to that described by Jackson affecting the caecum and ascending colon. As a rule this has no serious import, but in some cases where kinking of the ureter is found—particularly in association with prolapsed kidney—it may take on a more serious significance, fixing the ureter in an abnormal position and giving rise to severe renal crises with the formation of a hydronephrosis. Ureteric calculi may become impacted at an acute kink caused by one of these adhesions, and attacks of severe colic result.

Diagnosis. Attacks of pain in the kidney—not severe enough to merit the term colic—accompanied by urinary infection and slight pelvic dilatation should raise the suspicion of ureteric adhesions. This will be strengthened if there is no evidence of stone in the X-ray, and if the pyelogram by Abrodil or retrograde method shows marked ureteral kinking and dilatation.

Treatment. Treatment consists in exposing the kidney and ureter in the loin, removing any membrane-like adhesions which may be present, and by means of a nephropexy elevating and fixing the kidney, thereby straightening the ureter in its abdominal course.

CALCULUS

Calculi in the ureter have usually been previously manufactured in the kidney. Occasionally they may represent particles of a large branching renal calculus which have become detached and extruded from the renal pelvis. Generally oval in shape, they resemble a date stone or revolver bullet. Rarely, they may be as large as a pigeon's egg. They pass down the ureter with successive attacks of colic, or become arrested at the upper or lower end, or at the site of an acute kink or adhesion. Dilatation of ureter and pelvis may be present above them.

Signs and Symptoms. Severe pain—paroxysmal and colicky in nature—is the most constant symptom, starting in the kidney, passing down the ureter, and often radiating to testis or labium.

The kidney is tender, and pain or discomfort along some part of the ureter is commonly found. Occasionally a small area corresponding with the position of the stone may be made

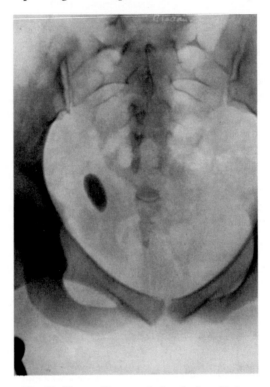

Fig. 21. X-ray of large ureteric calculus. (Later removed by operation.)

out, pressure on which elicits a pricking sensation. When the stone is impacted in the lower end of the ureter vesical symptoms such as urgency, frequency and strangury may develop. Haematuria, variable in amount, usually succeeds the pain. Rigidity of the abdominal wall and lumbar region on the affected side is commonly present during an attack.

Urinary infection of some degree usually makes its appearance within a few days. Slight rise of temperature is not uncommon.

The only urological conditions likely to be confused with calculus are intermittent hydronephrosis, or large blood clots descending the ureter from a kidney already the seat of growth or tubercle.

Intraperitoneal emergencies (e.g. appendicular, biliary or intestinal colic and obstruction) occasionally cause difficulty in the diagnosis.

Diagnosis. The provisional diagnosis of ureteric calculus is not, as a rule, difficult. Severe colic, together with a tender kidney and radiating pain—particularly if haematuria has occurred—will draw attention to the probability of this condition.

From the point of view of the general surgeon, exclusion of an intraperitoneal complaint is essential, and must generally be based on the clinical conditions alone. The more specialized investigation of the urologist will usually take place when colic has ceased.

Radiology is most helpful, and a characteristic shadow in the line of the ureter almost diagnostic. Shadows of calculi, however, may be confused with calcareous deposits in glands or veins, and some calculi are not opaque to the X-rays and therefore not shown in the skiagram.

Cystoscopy as a rule will be necessary. Stones at the lower end of the ureter may be visible, or the marked oedema—often bullous in nature—surrounding the ureteric orifice may indicate their presence.

Calculi situated higher up, may often be localized and demonstrated by a combination of radiology and cystoscopy.

An opaque ureteric bougie is introduced through the

cystoscope and passed up the ureter until its point is arrested, when the skiagram is taken. This method is most useful in confirming the nature of shadows which, either by their shape or position, raise doubt as to their interureteric nature.

Occasionally, where there is strong reason to suppose a calculus is present although radiology is negative, it may be helpful to pass a wax-tipped bougie guarded during its introduction through the cystoscope by a celluloid shield. This latter is detached in the bladder and the wax-tipped bougie introduced into the ureter. Scratches on the wax indicate the presence of a ureteric calculus.

Treatment. Many of the smaller ureteric calculi are passed naturally. After successive attacks of colic, with a lower and lower localization of pain, the calculus is felt to slip into the bladder and later to be extruded at micturition.

During an attack morphia and atropine should be given freely to relieve pain and spasm. Copious draughts of water and cherry-stalk tea are to be encouraged, and warmth in the form of fomentations or hot-water bottles may be applied to the abdomen and loin.

There is no contraindication to cystoscopy during an attack, although it is usually deferred until this has subsided. The passage of a small calculus may be considerably assisted by the injection into the ureter of a mixture of cocaine and almond oil which, by its lubricating and anaesthetic effects, often enables the calculus to be passed into the bladder a short time afterwards.

On the subsidence of an attack, if the stone is not too large, attempts should be made to encourage its passage *per vias naturales*. A calculus impacted in the lower end of the ureter may be freed either by incising the ureteric orifice with cystoscopic scissors, or by means of a ureterotome designed for use with the diathermic current. It may be extracted with cystoscopic forceps—or at least assisted into the bladder.

In the case of a more highly placed stone, dilatation of the ureter by means of bougie, or expanding dilator, together with its frequent lubrication may be helpful in assisting natural expulsion. Such methods should be given an extended trial before resorting to more heroic methods, unless calculus anuria has supervened.

Operative interference will be necessary:

(1) When cystoscopic methods have failed and calculous anuria is present.

(2) When calculi are adjudged too large to be passed naturally.

(3) When dilatation of the renal pelvis is commencing.

In these cases operation and extraction of the stone through the loin or the iliac fossa will be called for.

OPERATIONS

Two types of operation on the ureter are commonly performed:

(1) Ureteral lithotomy.

(2) Ureteral transplantation.

(1) Ureteral lithotomy may be practised either in the upper or lower part of the ureter.

(a) In the upper part the approach is the same as that for exposure of the kidney (q.v.).

(b) The approach to the ureter at the pelvic brim or in the pelvis is effected through a curved incision similar to that for extraperitoneal ligature of the common iliac artery. Its extent will vary with the size and fatness of the individual but will usually be $4\frac{1}{2}$ in. long. Skin, fascia, and aponeurosis of the external oblique muscle are severed in the line of incision.

The internal oblique and transversalis muscles may be split horizontally in the line of their fibres, or—if extra space is needed—in the line of the original incision, without damaging the anterior abdominal wall to any extent.

When the peritoneum is reached, this is pushed inwards until the pelvic brim and external iliac artery are defined. If stripping of the peritoneum is carried further, the ureter will adhere to it and can be easily identified as a prominent ridge exhibiting vermicular contractions on stimulation by gentle stroking or pinching. It can be detached from the posterior aspect of the peritoneum, and a hook or piece of tape passed round it to act as a retractor. From this point it can be traced upwards or downwards, care being taken to leave its blood supply intact.

When the contained calculus is localized the ureter may be incised either superficial to it or, if more convenient, at some distance from it, its edges held apart by tenacula, and the stone extracted by means of curved forceps. The ureter may be repaired, after verifying the patency of its vesical end by insertion of a probe.

If much sepsis is present it is advisable to drain the ureter by means of a small red-rubber catheter introduced through its wound—similar in practice to the drainage of the hepatic duct after the removal from it of stones.

If the opening from the ureter is repaired, an eyeless intestinal needle with No. 00 catgut is advisable—care being taken to see that stenosis is not produced. Insertion of a rubber drain down to the opening is essential. The wound is closed in successive layers, and the drain removed on the fourth day unless much urine is escaping. If a catheter has been inserted in the ureter it should be withdrawn on the seventh day.

(2) The transplantation of ureters from bladder to bowel may be called for in:

(*a*) Ectopia vesicae, and epispadias.

(*b*) Certain types of vesical and ureteral fistula.

(*c*) Growth of the bladder.

(*d*) Severe vesical ulceration with contracted ("systolic") bladder.

Before embarking on this procedure it is essential for the operator to appreciate two fundamental principles:

(i) A valve-like opening from ureter to bowel must be fashioned in order to replace the normal sphincteric mechanism between ureter and bladder, and thereby prevent infection ascending to the kidneys.

(ii) Efficient renal secretion must be maintained.

These two conditions are to a certain extent antagonistic in their demands, for if no attempt is made to construct a "uretero-colic" sphincter, urinary secretion will be unimpeded, but dilatation and ascending infection will supervene. Conversely, if an efficient sphincter is constructed by the formation of an oblique passage through the bowel wall, protection against infection is adequate, but renal secretion may be temporarily prevented by inflammatory exudate and swelling at the junction of ureter and bowel.

In order to comply with these two essentials, a "uretero-colic" sphincter is formed by making a channel between the sero-muscular and mucous coats of the bowel in which the ureter is embedded for an inch or more before finally perforating the mucous membrane to open into the lumen of the gut. To ensure sufficient urinary excretion, transplantation of each ureter is carried out at separate times with an interval of 14–21 days between, or if both ureters be transplanted at a single sitting, ureteric catheters can be introduced into their lumena and allowed to project through the rectum, thereby ensuring a patent channel for the passage of urine.

Technique. The abdomen is opened and the patient placed in a fairly steep Trendelenberg position. The pelvis is emptied of coils of intestine by pushing them upwards into the abdomen and retaining them there by abdominal pads. The right ureter is first sought and easily identified as it crosses the pelvic brim behind the peritoneum. This latter is incised and dissected off the ureter to within about an inch of its

termination. The ureter is gently freed from its bed, care
being taken not to strip it unnecessarily or impair its rather
slender blood supply. A hook or narrow tape placed under it
acts as an admirable retractor when necessary.

The lower part of the sigmoid is then sought for, a longitudinal muscle band (tenia) identified, and an area 2–3 in.
long just to the side of the tenia is grasped at either end by
a pair of vulsellum forceps. By gentle traction on the vulsella
the serous coat is rendered taut between them and is incised
for a distance of $1\frac{1}{2}$ in., care being taken not to open the
mucous membrane.

The ureter is now cut across as low down as possible, the
vesical end ligatured, and the proximal end grasped in the
points of a vulsellum or dissecting forceps. It is trimmed into
the form of a pen-nib, and an intestinal needle threaded with
No. 0 catgut passed through the point of the nib-shaped
extremity and gently tied, leaving a 3 in. "short end" which,
by means of a probe, is insinuated into the lumen of the
ureter to act as a "catgut guide" for the urine. The long end
attached to the needle is then taken by an assistant. The
surgeon next makes a stab wound through the mucous
membrane at the lower end of the gutter previously fashioned
in the sigmoid. Through this stab wound is passed the
intestinal needle which, after entering the lumen of the
sigmoid, is then made to pierce its walls and reappear about
an inch beyond the lower extremity of the sero-mucous gutter.

By traction on its catgut, the ureter is pulled into the bowel
and a partial fixation is effected by passing the needle once
or twice through the serous coat to form a ligature. Another
intestinal needle then buries the terminal inch of the ureter
in the bowel wall by uniting the incision in the sero-muscular
coat outside the duct. These stitches should pass through the
anterior wall of the ureter to assist its retention in position.
The opening in the posterior peritoneum is then closed.

The left ureter is generally to be found lying lateral to the sigmoid, and is similarly transplanted at a slightly different level either into the longitudinal tenia or to the left of it some 14 days later.

If both ducts are to be transplanted at the same time, ureteric catheters are introduced into the ureters immediately after their severancy. The catheters pass through sigmoid, rectum and anus to the outside, and by preventing compression of the ureteral lumen by inflammatory exudates, thereby prevent a dangerous or fatal anuria.

Chapter VII

THE BLADDER

ANATOMY AND PHYSIOLOGY

From the surgical point of view the **male bladder** may be looked on as a hollow muscle, arranged in three layers—an inner and outer longitudinal, and an intermediate circular layer well marked at the bladder outlet to form a sphincter. These are lined by an internal mucous membrane.

The bladder is divided into a body, a base or trigone looking towards the rectum, an apex towards the symphysis pubis, and a neck which is continued into the urethra and surrounded by the prostate. The upper surface and the posterior surface as low as the ureters is covered with peritoneum. From these surfaces this structure passes backwards to the rectum, laterally to the side walls of the pelvis, and anteriorly to the abdominal wall forming the false ligaments of the bladder. The true ligaments are condensed strands of pelvic fascia connecting the bladder with pubis, side walls of the pelvis, and sacrum. The anterior wall of the bladder is devoid of peritoneum, brown and ridged in appearance, and is covered with tortuous veins making it easily recognizable in the operation of suprapubic cystotomy.

The interior of the bladder, when inspected by the cystoscope, consists of two distinct parts—an upper (the body) and a lower (the trigone). The body possesses a loosely attached mucous membrane, often rugose, and trabeculation may be present varying with age and the degree of obstruction to urinary outflow. Small or large pouches may occur between the trabeculae. The trigone, or base, is bounded by the three openings of right and left ureter and urethra.

The ureters are placed on well-marked ridges, and their normal orifices may be slit-like, circular, or horseshoe shaped.

The interureteric bar (of Mercier) is sometimes prominent. The mucous membrane is tightly attached to the trigone, is smooth, and non-rugose. It is usually of a slightly deeper pink than that of the body of the bladder.

Sphincteric and Nervous Mechanism

The outlet from the bladder is surrounded by a concentration of its circular plain muscle fibres to form the so-called internal sphincter. A fan-shaped muscle (the trigonal muscle) passing from the interureteric ridge above the sphincter is inserted into the posterior lip of the urethra. The external sphincter is to all intents and purposes the sphincter urethrae membranaceae surrounding the membraneous urethra. These three muscles are intimately concerned with the normal act of micturition.

The nerve supply of the bladder is derived from three sources:

(1) Lumbar (sympathetic).
(2) Sacral (parasympathetic).
(3) Pudic (to external sphincter).

The lumbar innervation consists of fibres derived from the second and third lumbar sympathetic ganglia, together with branches from the pre-aortic and inferior mesenteric plexus. These fibres are concentrated into a narrow ribbon-like strand, passing in front of the bifurcation of the aorta, the left common iliac vein, and the fifth lumbar vertebra, and nowadays usually called the presacral nerve. This nerve lies in front of the midsacral artery, and, in front of the sacral promontory, divides into two pelvic plexuses from which fibres are carried to the bladder. They are usually considered to be inhibitory to the body, and motor to the sphincter (the "filling" nerves).

The parasympathetic supply consists of fibres derived from the second, third, and fourth sacral nerves, and these reach the bladder as the pelvic nerves. They convey motor impulses to the body and inhibit the sphincter (the "emptying" nerves). Running with both these motor supplies are sensory fibres. This latter point is worthy of note as it is not an uncommon experience for a surgeon who has administered a low spinal anaesthetic, with successful blocking of the sacral nerves, to find a considerable degree of sensibility in the prostate or bladder base—signifying the escape of the higher lumbar centre from anaesthetization.

Branches from the pudic nerve (S. II, III, and IV) supply the striated muscles of the perineum including the sphincter urethrae membranaceae—sometimes referred to as the external sphincter.

Micturition is effected in three phases. Firstly, the trigonal muscle pulling back the posterior lip of the internal urinary meatus allows a few drops of urine to enter the upper urethra. The stimulation of this "trigger area" next inhibits the sphincter vesicae, and lastly a powerful contraction of the body results in a voiding of the bladder contents.

The lymphatic drainage of the bladder is to the external, internal, and common iliac glands.

Female Bladder. This differs only slightly from the male, being rather smaller and somewhat pyriform in shape. It is intimately connected with the lower part of the uterus and upper part of the vagina, and the peritoneum passes from its upper surface directly to the anterior aspect of the uterus.

PATHOLOGY

Pathological changes in the vascular supply of the bladder may take the form of hyperaemia, anaemia, haemorrhage and oedema. These conditions can be recognized by cystoscopy and the following points are worthy of note:

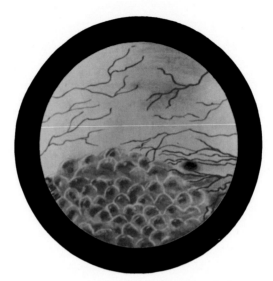

Fig. 22. Cystoscopic View of Bullous Oedema

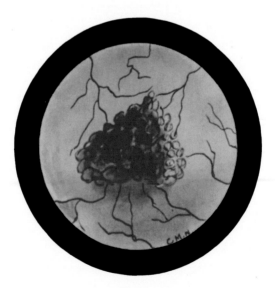

Fig. 23. Cystoscopic View of Papilloma of Bladder

Hyperaemia may be active (arterial), or passive (venous). Active hyperaemia is generally due to irritation produced by drugs or micro-organisms. Pregnancy is an additional cause. It is found in cystitis when a large area of the bladder may be affected, or it may be localized around the orifice of one or both ureters in renal tuberculosis. Swollen and engorged vessels may be present at the opening of one ureter in cases of renal growth, but it is unjustifiable to assume the presence of a growth on this sign alone. Passive or venous hyperaemia is evidenced by a cyanotic area, with swelling of the surrounding tissue, and is generally due to thrombosis, or to the pressure of a pregnant uterus or pelvic tumour.

Anaemia. Anaemic areas in the bladder mucosa are not common and, unless very white, are not easy to identify with the cystoscope. They are due to compression of the arterial supply from some extravesical cause.

Haemorrhage. Local haemorrhage and extravasation appear as a darkish patch on the surface of the bladder, or small bleeding areas may sometimes be seen.

Oedema. Oedema is not uncommon. The surface of the mucous membrane is raised, and usually pale and glossy in appearance. Occasionally polypoid excrescences are present. The commonest cause is a stone impacted at the lower end of the ureter, although it may also be present in inflammatory or malignant affections in and around the bladder.

Bullous oedema. This curious condition is very characteristic, and easily identified. It consists of numerous bullae arranged like cobblestones, usually of a pink or reddish colour, and most commonly found in the region of the trigone, although it may occur in any part of the bladder mucosa. The area is definitely outlined, raised and covered by a smooth glistening epithelium. When it occurs it is usually associated with an intense cystitis, intestino-vesical fistula, tubercle, or carcinoma of the uterus or prostate (Fig. 22). To sum up, oedema and inflammation surrounding a ureteric orifice generally denote ureteric stone, tubercle or inflammation of the kidney of that side. Hyperaemia, alone, of a ureteric orifice may be present in cases of renal tumour, or after a profuse haemorrhage from that side.

MALFORMATIONS

ECTOPIA VESICAE (Extroversion)

This distressing condition results from an absence of the front of the bladder and the anterior abdominal wall. It is associated with incomplete development of the pubic bones and failure to form a symphysis, epispadias, and usually undescended testes. Below the navel a patch of mucous membrane is visible with the openings of the two ureters from which urine is continually ejected. The skin round about is sodden, and often excoriated, and the patient's life a misery owing to continual soaking of his clothes, smell and ulceration.

Treatment. In the past this has been unsatisfactory, as attempts to perform plastic operations in this region have invariably failed or, at best, have resulted in the formation of a reservoir devoid of sphincteric control. Nowadays, only one type of treatment is to be advocated, that of ureteral transplantation into the sigmoid which should be carried out as early as possible. About 6 years of age will be found the earliest suitable time at which to operate, and after the transplantation of the second ureter the ectopic bladder may be excised and a plastic operation performed to close the gap in the abdominal wall. This latter may be extremely difficult, and not always advisable. (For details of ureteral transplantation see under chapter VI.)

DIVERTICULA

Diverticula of the bladder are not uncommon. They are generally situated on the lateral or posterior wall. They vary considerably in size, and have a well-marked rounded opening into the bladder. Their contents may become infected, and calculi may develop therein. Their presence may be suspected in cases of intractable cystitis for which no adequate cause can be found. They may give rise to frequency, and occasionally urine is passed in two parts—the first being comparatively clear, the second markedly purulent. Diagnosis is by means of the cystoscope, their size being calculated by the passage of ureteric catheters into their lumen, or by means of a cystogram.

Treatment will depend on size and infection of their contents. In the early stages lavage by means of a ureteric catheter introduced into their lumen through a cystoscope is advisable. After their contents have been washed out they may be filled with liquid paraffin, which, for a short time at least, prevents the accumulation in them of further pus. If possible they should be excised. If this method is not feasible, it may be possible to enlarge their opening into the bladder sufficiently to ensure their complete drainage.

RUPTURE

Rupture of the bladder is almost entirely confined to males. Apart from penetrating injuries (e.g. gunshot wounds and fracture of the pelvis) it is most likely to result from a kick or knock on the distended organ. Except from an ulcerated or cancerous bladder, spontaneous rupture is unknown. Rupture may be intra- or extraperitoneal, the former variety being the commoner.

Signs and Symptoms. There is the history of an injury, and shock is usually severe. Pain is present, and often an intense desire to pass water exists, although none can be voided. The lower part of the abdomen is rigid and tender, and bruising may be present. If a catheter is passed only a few drops of blood-stained urine are withdrawn. In extraperitoneal rupture extravasation of urine takes place into the pelvic connective tissue, and may track via the obturator and sciatic foramena into the thigh and buttock, or ascend along the anterior abdominal wall.

Diagnosis. Every case of fractured pelvis should be examined for signs of vesical rupture. Rupture of the urethra is the most likely condition to be confused with it, and where this rupture is in the posterior urethra diagnosis apart from operation may be impossible. Retention of urine may occur after pelvic fractures without a rupture of the bladder being present. The passage of a catheter will render the diagnosis clear, and should not be withheld.

Treatment. Treatment is urgent and operation should be carried out forthwith. If the rupture is intraperitoneal, closure of the rent may not be difficult after mopping out urine and blood from the abdomen. Drainage of the bladder, through a suprapubic tube preferably, or by means of an indwelling catheter, is necessary. Extraperitoneal rupture needs suprapubic cystotomy and drainage of the perivesical tissues, the rent being closed when possible. Areas to which extravasated urine may have permeated should be inspected daily, and on signs of infection becoming evident they should be incised and drained.

FOREIGN BODIES AND CALCULUS
FOREIGN BODIES

Various types of foreign body may be found in the bladder—hairpins, slate pencils and portions of catheters being the most frequent. They are more common in women than in men, and have, as a rule, been self-introduced. Rarely, foreign bodies may ulcerate into the bladder from other abdominal organs (e.g. gallstones or sequestra). Any foreign body may become incrusted with the urinary salts and form the nucleus of a calculus.

Symptoms. The symptoms most commonly present are frequency, pyuria and haematuria, with occasional bouts of retention. Routine examination with X-ray and cystoscope renders the diagnosis certain.

Treatment. If comparatively small they can be extracted through or together with the operating cystoscope by means of suitable forceps. If too large for this, suprapubic cystotomy will be called for.

CALCULUS

Bladder stones are usually rounded in appearance, generally free from facets and, though commonly single, several may be present. They are usually formed of uric acid, or urates of sodium or ammonium. Calcium oxalate is not uncommon, and phosphatic stones are frequent. Phosphatic stones are creamy white in appearance, uric acid stones yellowish and oxalic calculi dark brown.

Clinical Features. The patient, usually a man of middle age (although vesical calculus in infancy is not uncommon), complains of increased frequency of micturition, pain at the end of the penis after passing water and in the perineum after taking exercise. Pyuria may be present, and haematuria—often slight in amount—usually occurs at some time in the disease. He may give a history of urination being suddenly cut off, as by a tap, if the stone has occluded the internal urinary meatus. In advanced cases much pus may be present, and infection ascending to the kidneys may have given rise to rigors, high temperature and signs of renal impairment. Calculi may occur in a post-prostatic pouch, or in a diverticulum of the bladder, and are not uncommon in the prostatic cavity after prostatectomy.

Diagnosis. A skiagram will nearly always render the diagnosis obvious. A stone may be discovered by the cystoscope and, as a rule, presents no difficulties of recognition.

Occasionally, however, blood clots or sloughs left after the removal of a prostate may closely resemble small calculi. If there is doubt as to the nature of any foreign body in the bladder a ureteric catheter may be passed and the foreign body probed—a clot or slough may be broken up, and a stone dislodged and inspected from another aspect, when its identity may be revealed. Metal sounds, by the characteristic grating they afford to the examiner when the stone is touched, may be sufficient to effect a diagnosis, but they are not to be recommended when radiology and cystoscopy are possible. In the case of young children they may, however, be employed when a cystoscope of small enough calibre is not available.

Treatment. Two methods only in the treatment of vesical calculi need be considered:

(1) Litholapaxy—or crushing of the stone.
(2) Lithotomy—or the removal of the stone unbroken through a suprapubic opening.

In rare cases, however, where very small stones are present and are not voided naturally, they may be extracted with the aid of the operating cystoscope *per urethram*. In adults litholapaxy is, in most cases, the method of choice. It is, however, contraindicated in the following conditions:

(*a*) Severe sepsis.
(*b*) Encystment of the stone.
(*c*) Excessive hardness of the stone.
(*d*) Extremely small urethrae—as in children—or where stricture is present.

Before its employment a previous cystoscopy must have been carried out to determine the shape, size, and characteristics of the calculus, and the operation then performed by means of a cystoscopic lithotrite. Where litholapaxy is impracticable, lithotomy will become necessary. Nowadays—in England at least—it is invariably carried out via the suprapubic route.

CYSTITIS

Cystitis may be acute or chronic, and is caused by a variety of organisms—of which the commonest is the *B. coli communis*—in association with lowered vitality of the bladder. Infection may be acquired via the urethra (less commonly than was formerly supposed), or by means of a downward travel from kidney and ureter (by far the commonest route). A *primary* cystitis is practically unknown, and it cannot be too much emphasized that the diagnosis of cystitis alone is usually unjustified and misleading.

Since micro-organisms may traverse the bladder for long periods without giving rise to a cystitis, it is generally held that the presence in the bladder, or its neighbourhood, of some abnormal condition is necessary. This, by lowering the vitality of the bladder, renders it liable to infection from the urine. Such predisposing causes may take the form of calculi, or foreign bodies. Enlargement of the prostate and stricture, by preventing effective emptying of the bladder with the consequent retention of residual urine, may become potent factors.

Bacteria, which descend from the kidney and would normally be excreted without comment on the part of the urological system, find in the abraded mucous membrane of the bladder already housing a stone, or in the stagnant urine behind an enlarged prostate, a suitable medium in which to develop.

In certain cases micro-organisms may be introduced into the bladder on unclean instruments. In other cases carefully sterilized instruments may traverse a urethra infected with the gonococcus or other bacteria, thereby introducing it into the bladder. In yet other cases, gonococci may extend directly from urethra to bladder.

The commonest organisms giving rise to cystitis—as has already been mentioned—are of the *B. coli* group, but staphylococci are not uncommon, while streptococci, enterococci, *B. proteus* and others are found from time to time.

Pathologically the condition consists of a well-marked injection of the vessels of the mucous membrane, usually most severe in the region of the trigone. Bleeding points may be visible and, as infection increases, oedema and ulceration may make their appearance. Pus is present, and in chronic cases may be profuse.

Clinically the signs and symptoms will vary in severity with the acuteness of the condition and the intensity of the infection. Frequency is always present in some degree, and the passage of urine may have to be effected as often as every 20 min. in extreme cases. The amount of urine passed at each act is always small. It may contain blood in fair quantity, or a few drops only may be extruded at the end of micturition. Pus is an invariable constituent. The reaction of the urine may be acid or alkaline. It is usually the latter, but in certain early cases of *B. coli* infection it may be acid. In later cases of *B. coli* infection, and where urinary stagnation is present, the reaction will be alkaline. It may become foul smelling and ammoniacal on standing. Pain is always present in the acute condition but may be absent in the more chronic types. It may take the form of three varieties which probably indicate a difference in the pathological condition in the bladder.

(1) Pain may be present at the beginning or ending of micturition—referred to the penis. (This probably indicates a severe trigonitis without gross ulceration.)

(2) It may take the form of an intense straining—the whole urethra feeling as if it were on fire—associated with severe spasm of the bladder musculature. [Strangury. This probably

denotes a more advanced condition than that previously described, associated with ulceration of the bladder neck. It is conceivable that the spasmodic contraction of the bladder is an attempt to rid itself of the painful stimulation of the denuded area.]

(3) A much less severe type of pain, of the nature of an aching together with a feeling of weight, may be present in the perineum. (It probably indicates engorgement—if not infection—of the prostate rather than of the bladder itself.) Occasionally in men, and more commonly in women, pain and tenderness may be present above the pubis.

Some degree of temperature is present in the acute cases. In chronic cystitis it may not be raised at all, while high fevers and rigors indicate renal infection.

Diagnosis. The triad, pain, frequency, and pyuria, is sufficient on which to base a diagnosis. It cannot, however, be overstressed that it is the primary cause of cystitis that should be sought, rather than the diagnosis of an obvious condition. Where an acute inflammation—as evidenced by severe pain and rise of temperature—is present, it is inadvisable, in the early stages at least, to resort to instrumentation, and some degree of treatment may be necessary before a full investigation can be carried out. A skiagram of the urinary tract may be taken as soon as convenient. Cystoscopy should be deferred until the more acute symptoms have subsided. The chemical reaction of the urine may be helpful if acidity is noted, in that it suggests *B. coli* or tuberculosis as a causal agent. A specimen of urine passed into a clean vessel may be examined for the nature of the infective agent, but a catheter should not be introduced at this stage. On the subsidence of the acute symptoms, if the radiological examination has been negative, cystoscopy may be proceeded with, and a more effective bacteriological examination of the urine carried out.

The following conditions should be sought for and if found remedied:

(1) Gonorrhoeal urethritis. (The discovery of which should preclude the passage of a catheter or cystoscope.)
(2) Urethral stricture.
(3) Enlargement of the prostate.
(4) Cystocele in women.
(5) Vesical ulceration. (If not due to the presence of foreign bodies or calculi, is almost always associated with a descending infection from the kidneys of *B. coli* or tuberculosis.)
(6) Intestino-vesical fistula.

Treatment. The treatment is carried out in two phases:

(1) The treatment of symptoms in the acute stage.
(2) The remedying of the predisposing causes when the acute stage has passed.

Acute cystitis should be treated by copious draughts of barley water or cherry-stalk tea. A mixture containing 10 to 15 minims of the tincture of hyoscyamus, 15 grains of potassium citrate, and infusion of buchu, may help in the allaying of the spasmodic pain. Hot baths, and fomentations to the abdominal wall and perineum, also play their part. If the urine remains strongly acid steps should be taken to alter this reaction by the administration of larger doses of some alkali.

If there is any difficulty in rendering the urine alkaline, hexamine in 10 grain doses four times a day may be tried, as this acts only in an acid medium and in some cases may be the quickest way of destroying the bacteria.

In most sub-acute or chronic conditions, or where a post-operative cystitis exists, the urine is alkaline. In such cases attempts may be made to render it acid by the administration of ammonium benzoate, or acid sodium phosphate (gr xv–gr xxv t.d.s.) and when this is accomplished hexamine gr xv t.d.s. may be given. The newer drugs pyridium, neotropine and acriflavine may be helpful on occasion. Yet other cases may be benefited by cystopurin, or the intravenous injection of cylotropin.

Where pus is a marked feature, bladder washes of oxycyanide 1–6000, or silver nitrate solution 1–2000 rising to 1–500 may be helpful. If there is much pain the milder bladder washes of boracic, potassium permanganate and hydrogen peroxide may prove beneficial. No hard and fast rule can be laid down for the treatment of every case of chronic cystitis, but from personal experience the writer has found considerable benefit result from the use of neotropine, or pyridium, unless much mucus is secreted, in which case cystopurin is very often effective.

The intravenous injection of 5 c.c. of cylotropin on every other day is particularly helpful in clearing up a post-operative residual cystitis, especially if it is combined with four hourly 20 grain doses of ammonium benzoate. Excessively foul urines may often be rendered comparatively clean by increasingly strong bladder washes of silver nitrate.

Occasionally, a persistently septic urine resists all the more conservative types of treatment, and it may become necessary to perform a suprapubic cystotomy to effect adequate drainage. This is sometimes necessary as a preliminary stage in the removal of the prostate, both to clear up a cystitis and to relieve stress on the kidneys.

TUBERCULOUS CYSTITIS
See under chapter ix (Urinary tuberculosis).

FISTULA
Three types of vesical fistula occur:
>   (1) Suprapubic.
>   (2) Intestino-vesical.
>   (3) Vesico-vaginal.

(1) Suprapubic Vesical Fistula

Rarely, the persistence of the foetal allantois after birth may leave a small track between the bladder and umbilicus, discharging urine. It may be present in an otherwise normal infant, or in association with an occluded urethra in which case it acts as a safety valve. If the urethral outlet from the bladder is normal the fistulous track may be excised. The commonest cause of a suprapubic fistula is the non-healing of a cystotomy wound due to obstruction at the bladder neck (e.g. post-prostatectomy contraction, calculi or highly septic urine). The presence of a pouch, or diverticulum, with septic contents can also be a responsible factor.

Treatment consists in removing the causes indicated. Curettage, or excision of the track may be necessary later.

(2) Intestino-vesical Fistula

This is not very uncommon. It is much more frequent in men than in women, and may take place between bladder and sigmoid, rectum, caecum, appendix or small intestine. Adhesion between bowel and bladder, as the result of inflammatory or malignant disease, with the breaking down of the partition between them on the bursting of the abscess, or extension of the malignant disease, is the causal factor. When affecting the sigmoid or rectum, carcinoma or diverticulitis is the commonest cause, but an abscess which has burst into the bladder may communicate by its other extremity with the caecum, appendix, or sigmoid colon.

The opening is usually on the posterior wall or vertex. Pneumaturia is the first symptom, rapidly followed by the development of a cystitis. Faeces may appear in the urine, either intermittently, or continuously: when the small intestine is affected they will resemble the contents of the ileum—being yellowish in colour. When the large bowel is at fault they will be darker brown in tint and more solid in consistence. Cystoscopically a patch of intense cystitis—often surrounded by bullous oedema—is visible. The opening of the fistula plugged by faeces may be seen, although it is more frequently masked by the surrounding oedema.

Diagnosis is usually easy, but the particular part of the bowel affected may not be determined until operation is undertaken.

Treatment. If it is due to an old appendix abscess the condition may heal spontaneously. The removal of the appendix—if present—and the freeing of the caecum if the fistula persists should, however, be undertaken without undue delay.

If the left colon is affected, bladder and colonic lavage should be instigated. Occasionally a cure will result. More commonly the condition will persist with some amelioration of the cystitis.

Operation in these cases is generally inadvisable. When a carcinoma of the colon has invaded the bladder, complete removal may not be feasible, and the fistulous channel may be of the nature of a safety valve preventing acute intestinal obstruction. Furthermore, in both malignant disease of the colon and where diverticulitis is the causal agent, the performance of a colostomy alone merely effects the substitution of an external for an internal fistula—a consummation not always to be desired on the part of the patient. Nevertheless, each case must be judged on its merits and where, after due consideration of the history and examination by means of barium enemata and X-rays, there is reason to suppose that the intestinal and vesical tracts can be satisfactorily separated, operation should be undertaken. It is, however, likely to be difficult and the shock severe, owing to the presence of numerous adhesions, and until the interior of the abdomen has been inspected no one can foretell the chances of success.

(3) Vesico-vaginal Fistula

This rarely occurs apart from damage to the bladder at operation, or parturition. The continued escape of decomposing urine from the vagina draws attention to the condition. Cystoscopy shows the vesical end of the fistula, as a rule, without difficulty. A ureteric catheter can be passed through this opening into the vagina, thus demonstrating its position in that organ, where it may have been difficult to identify.

Treatment consists in rendering the urine as clean as possible. This may necessitate a preliminary cystotomy. A plastic operation, through bladder and vagina combined, should be undertaken when the urine is clear. Drainage of the bladder through the suprapubic route, or by an indwelling catheter, must be carried out for at least a week after operation.

GROWTHS OF BLADDER

Both innocent and malignant tumours of the bladder occur, but the two types tend to merge and clinically it is often impossible to differentiate between them.

Pathology. The so-called innocent papilloma, or villus tumour—originally single—often becomes multiple as the disease progresses, or after partial removal, when small "seedlings" may have been implanted in the mucous membrane. After total removal of one of these histologically benign growths, recurrence of a more malignant type is not uncommon. These neoplasms may be situated anywhere in the bladder; most commonly they occur just lateral to the trigone. The growth consists of a central core of fibrous, muscular and vascular tissues, which branch like the boughs of a tree and are covered by a transitional epithelium. Vesical papillomata, although possessing a marked tendency to recurrence after removal, and ability to seed themselves by implantation on apparently normal mucous membrane, do not produce metastases nor—in the early stages at least—do they invade the bladder wall to produce a perivesical spread (Fig. 23).

Malignant growths of the bladder occur in four distinct types:

        (1) Papillomatous.
        (2) Nodular.
        (3) Infiltrating.
        (4) Sarcomatous.

(1) The malignant papilloma resembles its more innocent brother fairly closely, but the villi are more stunted and the tumour is more likely to be sessile than pedunculated. Microscopically it is seen to be a carcinoma.

(2) The nodular, or "bald", growths are button-like excrescences, varying greatly in size. Villi are replaced by minute papillae and surface necrosis is common. Their base tends to infiltrate the bladder wall.

(3) The infiltrating growth takes the form of a flat plaque, or ulcer, with a wide spread in the bladder wall. All these malignant epithelial tumours usually remain localized to the bladder for a considerable time, but sooner or later they extend through its walls to the perivesical tissues and invade other organs (e.g. rectum or vagina). Fistulae may occur, but metastases in lymphatic glands and bones are rare.

(4) Rarely, sarcoma may occur. It usually arises from the submucous or perivesical connective tissue. The growth is sessile or pedunculated, and invasive in character. It tends to occur at the extremes of life.

Signs and Symptoms. Haematuria, at first painless—although later perhaps associated with frequency and some discomfort on passing water—is the most characteristic, and often the only sign of vesical growth. Small particles of the tumour may be detached and become visible in the urine. Bleeding with clot formation may be severe so that retention of urine may occur and the patient show signs of anaemia. As the growth enlarges cystitis develops, and calculi may be deposited on its surface. In the malignant, invasive type, considerable pain may be produced when ulceration exposes the deeper tissues, and frequency may become intense. Where a malignant growth is large, an abdominal tumour can sometimes be felt in the hypogastric region.

A vaginal or rectal examination may reveal considerable extravesical spread with fixity of the bladder even to the pelvic walls, or smaller palpable nodules may be present in the anterior rectal or vaginal wall. Renal efficiency may be much impaired if the growth is extensive and is obstructing the ureters.

Investigation, Diagnosis and Treatment must generally proceed hand in hand. The primary diagnosis is by means of the cystoscope, and though it may occasionally be difficult to identify the growth owing to the rapid clouding of the medium by blood, prolonged lavage will usually allow of a satisfactory—although rapid—inspection of the tumour.

Occasionally cystoscopy may have to be deferred until, or repeated after, bleeding has abated. A rectal or vaginal examination should never be omitted, as fixity of the bladder, extravesical masses, and nodular growths in bladder, vagina, or rectal wall, can thereby often be detected. Before satisfactory treatment can be initiated the following questions have to be answered:

       (1) What is the position of the tumour?
       (2) Is it innocent or malignant?
       (3) Is it removable?
       (4) If removable, what is the best method of
           effecting this?

(1) This can be settled by cystoscopy alone.

(2) The innocent growth is rarely larger than a walnut, but there may be more than one villus tumour present. The fringes are usually well marked and the growth or growths pedunculated and easy to identify and localize, as bleeding

during examination is easier to control than in the malignant types. Pain is generally absent.

Malignant growths are generally sessile with rudimentary or stumpy villi, and though often extensive are usually single. Bleeding is more difficult to control and pain is more commonly present.

(3) Innocent growths—particularly if small—are most effectively removed by perurethral diathermy. Equally, growths—innocent or malignant—which are situated in the vertex and do not encroach on the ureters can usually be removed by means of a partial cystectomy, unless a malignant extension to other viscera has occurred. When a growth is situated in close proximity to the ureters or is of large dimensions, removal may be very difficult apart from cystectomy. Malignant growths which have extended outside the bladder with fixity of that organ, or with the formation of a palpable tumour, are unsuitable for removal.

(4) Removal of intravesical growths may be carried out by means of:

(a) **Diathermy**—effected (i) through the cystoscope, or (ii) through a suprapubic opening.

(b) **Excision**, which should take the form of a partial cystectomy, thereby removing not only the growth itself but that part of the bladder wall from which it originates.

The older operation of excision carried out through a suprapubic wound and from the inside of the bladder may be necessary if the neoplasm is situated close to the ureters, or on the bladder base.

(c) **Total cystectomy**, after preliminary transplantation of the ureters, may be necessary for malignant or massive "innocent" growths.

It is obviously impossible to indicate in detail the treatment of bladder neoplasm in a work of this size, but the following brief epitome may be of help to those for whom this manual is designed:

(i) Diathermy carried out through the cystoscope is simple and efficacious in the treatment of innocent neoplasms, but totally useless when applied to malignant growths. It is therefore advisable to submit all small or moderate growths to this treatment on one or more occasions and note the result. It can be carried out under local anaesthesia of the urethra (as the growth is insensitive) at fortnightly intervals and the result observed. In most cases the growth shrinks rapidly and finally disappears, haemorrhage ceases, and a cure results. Several sittings may be necessary—dependent on the size of the growth and the calibre of the electrode used. The smaller growths can be treated through the ordinary catheterizing cystoscope, but the larger ones are more effectively dealt with through a cystoscope of operating or diathermic type carrying a heavier electrode.

In some cases a less desirable effect is produced, and after one or more sittings at each of which the growth has apparently been thoroughly coagulated, it is found at the subsequent examination to be no smaller—and indeed may appear larger. These growths, although appearing innocent to the eye, are undoubtedly malignant and further diathermy will be useless.

(ii) Solitary growths situated in the vertex should be excised together with the bladder wall giving them birth, if any suspicion of malignancy exists, or if of moderate size.

(iii) Growths situated on the anterior wall of the bladder and difficult to reach with the cystoscope, or large growths close to the trigone, are best dealt with through a suprapubic opening—either by means of excision, or by diathermy with a large electrode. Whether the removal of a growth is effected by excision or diathermy, the patient should be subjected to frequent cystoscopic review for many months. These vesical growths have a great tendency to recur, or small parts of them, detached at operation, may seed themselves in other parts of the bladder. Symptoms of a recurrence may be absent for a long time and the patient unaware of it until the growth, which may have reached very large proportions, gives rise to an extensive haematuria.

(iv) Massive growths involving a large part of the bladder lumen are most satisfactorily treated by total cystectomy. This operation, carried out after preliminary transplantation of the ureters, is by no means so mutilating nor the results so unsatisfactory as was generally held a few years ago. Even if, after ureteric transplantation, total cystectomy is not feasible, the patient's life is made far less miserable when relieved of the distressing pain, frequency and haemorrhage which was rapidly making existence intolerable. These patients soon learn to control their rectal micturition, which, after a short while, is not performed oftener than every 2 or 3 hours during the day or more than once or twice at night. The operation is within the competence of any good general surgeon, and the writer has never received anything but gratitude from those patients on whom it has been necessary to perform ureteric transplantation.

NERVOUS DISORDERS

Various spinal affections give rise to bladder signs—the most usual being tabes, but disseminated sclerosis, myelitis or cord injuries are additional factors.

The commonest vesical signs of nervous involvement are difficulty in micturition and retention of urine, although active or passive incontinence may afterwards take their place. Cystitis sooner or later makes its appearance, and upward spread of infection to the kidneys is often a terminal feature of these cases.

In tabes the cystoscopic appearance is often characteristic, showing well-marked trabeculation, although no visible obstruction is present.

Treatment consists in combating the infection, or preventing its appearance, and relieving retention by catheterization when it occurs.

Although the surgery of the sympathetic system is as yet in its extreme infancy, cases arise in which an overaction of its influences or an underaction of its antagonist—the parasympathetic—are daily becoming more prominent in the eyes of the medical public.

Occasionally difficulty in emptying the bladder has been found to be due to underaction of the parasympathetic (sacral) nerve supply. For example, severe trauma to the conus medullaris or cauda equina, when a whole, or part, of the "emptying" nervous mechanism of the bladder may be damaged or destroyed.

It is obvious that if the whole centre or sacral nerves II, III and IV on both sides were completely destroyed, micturition could not take place. If, however, the destruction is only partial, removal of the sympathetic, or "filling", nervous influences—lumbar II and III—may allow of effective action of the residual sacral fibres. Cases in which accidental damage to the vesical emptying mechanism occurs are not common, but some ten or more have been described.

Again, certain highly nervous individuals may present signs of great difficulty in micturition, and recurrent bouts of urinary retention without demonstrable cause, which have been considered on somewhat slender evidence to be due to overaction on the part of the parasympathetic supply.

In both these types of cases satisfactory results have been obtained by excision of the presacral nerve in front of the fifth lumbar vertebra. This is the "bottle neck" through which the filling influences reach the bladder, and on their diminution or removal the emptying mechanism of the para-sympathetic supply is allowed unhampered action.

Cases which have received considerable benefit from this physiological type of operation are those in which damage to the sacral nerves has resulted, e.g. in operative removal of the rectum for carcinoma, or motor-car accidents involving the lower part of the spinal cord. The value of sympathectomy in these instances is therefore worth bearing in mind.

Chapter VIII

OPERATIONS ON THE BLADDER

Two types of operation are commonly practised on the bladder:

(1) Suprapubic.
(2) Perurethral, by means of cystoscope or operating cysto-urethroscope.

The older method of approach to the bladder via the perineum is obsolete, and is not described here.

SUPRAPUBIC OPERATIONS

Three operations on the bladder are practised via the suprapubic route:

(a) Cystotomy (and cystostomy).
(b) Partial cystectomy.
(c) Total cystectomy.

(a) Cystotomy, by its name, implies incision and exploration of the bladder: cystostomy, the more or less permanent drainage of that organ. With few exceptions these two principles are combined in the same operation:

(i) To relieve acute retention of the urine, from prostatic or urethral cause.
(ii) To drain the bladder when much pus is present.
(iii) To relieve pressure symptoms on bladder, kidney and ureter.
(iv) For intravesical removal of growth by excision or diathermy.
(v) For removal of vesical calculus, foreign body, or prostate.

In rupture of the bladder, or prostatic urethra, exploration of the bladder with suprapubic drainage will generally be called for. The operation will differ slightly according to whether the surgeon desires to examine the inside of the bladder or not.

In cases of acute urinary retention, or as a preliminary drainage of the bladder antecedent to prostatectomy where vesical calculus is absent, the suprapubic introduction of a self-retaining catheter through a small wound is to be recommended. To effect this, if the organ is not already over-full, the bladder is distended with water, saline or mild antiseptic, via the urethral catheter.

A short midline incision below the umbilicus and close to the highest point of the vesical swelling is then made, and the two rectus muscles separated. The prevesical pouch of peritoneum must be pushed upwards and out of the way by gentle gauze dissection, and the bladder identified as a brownish coloured organ, with several tortuous, vertically directed veins coursing along its anterior surface.

Puncture of the bladder is then effected by means of a Kidd's trocar and introducer. This consists of a metal rod 18 in. long, with a $\frac{3}{4}$ in. blade at its lower extremity, which is introduced through a self-retaining catheter of the Mallacott type. The blade is made to perforate and project from the closed end of the catheter, which is tightly stretched along the rod and maintained in position by a lever at the proximal end. The glorified trocar and cannula thus formed is introduced through a suitable spot in the anterior wall of the bladder, and the rod and its blade withdrawn, leaving the catheter *in situ*—tightly gripped by the opening in the bladder. In suitable cases no urine escapes by the side of the catheter, the wound is kept dry and uninfected, and the bladder can be emptied slowly or at intervals by removing a spigot from the end of the catheter. If desired, the catheter may be connected to a tube leading the urine away to a bottle fixed to the side of the bed. As an additional precaution against premature removal of the tube a stitch may be passed through it, attaching it to the skin.

Simple though this operation is, care is needed to make certain that the catheter does not slip over the very small "shoulder" at junction of knife and rod, thereby retracting and leaving the knife alone to enter the bladder. As a precaution against this, some surgeons prefer to use a specially large trocar and cannula introducing a catheter through the cannula on withdrawal of the trocar. In either method the great advantage of the dry suprapubic wound devoid of leakage beside the catheter is attained.

Where exploration of the inside of the bladder, or the removal of some foreign body is called for, the operation is of slightly greater magnitude. The incision through skin and fascia is longer, but rarely exceeds $4\frac{1}{2}$ in. The recti are separated, the peritoneum retracted upwards, and the bladder identified and incised. Urine will immediately escape, but a finger inserted into the cystotomy wound will prevent its too precipitate exit, and it is most satisfactorily removed from the operation area by the temporary introduction of a long and large calibre rubber tube. When most of the urine has escaped and the tube has been removed, the opening in the bladder is hooked up by the index finger of the left hand, and the edges of the wound are grasped by vulsellum forceps (or a catgut suture may be introduced on either side to act as a retractor). The wound in the bladder can be enlarged downwards if necessary, and the interior exposed by means of suitable retraction. Stones and foreign bodies can usually be removed by finger or forceps without the aid of visual inspection.

If it is desired to remove a papilloma situated in the lower part of the bladder through the transvesical route, or to subject it to diathermy, a self-retaining retractor should be introduced into the bladder, when the whole of its interior can be inspected. Removal may be carried out by cutting round its base, though haemorrhage may be considerable and can rarely be controlled by ligature. The application of the diathermy electrode is, however, easy, and in the opinion of the writer gives at least as good results as intravesical removal. The bladder is closed from below upwards, round a rubber tube at the uppermost point of the incision. This position of the tube will ensure a more rapid healing of the bladder than one more lowly placed, as escape through this opening is against gravity.

Furthermore, if another operation has to be carried out through the bladder (e.g. prostatectomy) this organ can be incised *below* the cystotomy wound without danger of opening the peritoneal sac. A small rubber drain should, however, be left in the pouch of Retzius on the closure of the anterior abdominal wall, to allow an effective exit for the products of sepsis in this region consequent on the spilling of urine.

Occasionally it may be necessary to open the bladder after traversing the peritoneal sac. Cases in which the bladder is much contracted, or to which peritoneum is tightly attached along the anterior wall as a result of previous operation and scarring in this region, are the types in which this will be necessary. Every precaution to exclude the general peritoneal cavity by suitable packs and close suture of the bladder wall around its drainage tube must be adopted.

(b) Partial cystectomy is called for in cases of malignant or suspicious growth involving the bladder walls above the level of the ureters.

The growth having previously been localized by cystoscopy, the bladder is moderately distended with boracic or oxy-cyanide solution. If the growth is situated in close proximity to a ureter, it is well as a preliminary to introduce a ureteric catheter into it by means of the cystoscope, as this can easily be identified by touch during the progress of the operation.

The patient is placed on his back, and an incision through the skin and fascia is made from umbilicus to pubis. The recti are well separated, the peritoneum dissected off the front and side walls of the bladder and pushed upwards to the vertex where the median umbilical ligament (the remains of the urachus) is tightly attached to it. This can be severed between ligatures, after which peritoneal separation proceeds easily.

If the growth is situated in the anterior wall or fundus of the bladder, the peritoneal stripping need not be carried very far back; but not uncommonly it must be proceeded with until the superior vesical vessels or ureters make their appearance. Not uncommonly the artery and vein will need division between ligatures.

It is here that the presence of a ureteric catheter, previously placed *in situ*, may be invaluable for the easy identification of the ureter. The growth can usually be palpated, and it is generally advisable to insert a suture at the lowest point beyond the growth to which cuts encircling the incision are likely to extend, as this materially helps in the suturing of the lower part of the wound. The growth is then excised, together with the bladder wall from which it springs, by a circumscribing incision half an inch or more from its base.

If peritoneum is involved in the spread of the tumour it must first be excised from the peritoneal sac, the opening of which should be closed before removal of the growth from the bladder is attempted.

Occasionally the growth is not palpable through the bladder wall, and an incision through the vesical vault may be necessary before it can be localized. The growth having been removed, closure—whole or partial—of the opening in the bladder should be carried out. In any case, drainage both of the bladder and of the perivesical space for a few days is necessary.

Vesical drainage will usually be carried out through the

wound of excision in that organ, but if the growth is situated to the posterior aspect it may be more convenient to close the wound of excision entirely, draining the bladder through a stab wound in its anterior wall.

In a few cases (e.g. in small growths of the vertex attended by slight haemorrhage and uninfected urine) it is justifiable to close the bladder completely, leaving a rubber drain down to its wall, and rely on an indwelling catheter to empty the bladder of its contents for 5 or 6 days.

Where from previous cystoscopy, or at the time of operation, malignant involvement of a single ureter is discovered, partial cystectomy may be carried out after the previous transplantation of this ureter into the sigmoid or vesical remnant.

(c) Total cystectomy is called for in malignant disease at the base of the bladder or involving both ureters. Very large innocent growths, or multiple papillomata with excessive haemorrhage, may require it for their successful extirpation. It is a much more severe operation than that previously described under partial cystectomy. One or more previous operations will have been necessary for the transplantation of the ureters into the sigmoid colon, and scarring may be considerable.

Total cystectomy can, as a rule, be carried out 14 days after the transplantation of the second ureter, or 3 weeks after the previous operation if both ureters were transplanted at the same sitting. This rough guide is based on the assumption that the patient's general condition is such as to render a severe operation not unduly hazardous.

A catheter is passed and the bladder moderately distended with fluid. The catheter is left *in situ* and clamped, or a wooden spigot is introduced into its open end. A midline incision from umbilicus to pubis, or even longer, is made through skin and fasciae of the anterior abdominal wall. The rectus muscles are separated, or if this does not give sufficient access, they may be detached from their insertion into the pubis. The peritoneum is then dissected from the bladder, to assist which, division of the median umbilical ligament is necessary.

At this stage the patient is placed in the Trendelenburg position, and stripping of the peritoneum proceeded with until the vesical vessels and ureters are defined. The vessels are divided between ligatures, and the ureters—already only short stumps—can usually be freed without much difficulty from the perivesical tissues. It is now that the bladder may be wholly or partially emptied by removing the spigot from the catheter. The writer prefers to empty the bladder completely at this stage and withdraw the catheter. The contracted and flaccid bladder is then grasped by suitable forceps and pulled up into the wound. The vesiculae seminales and vas deferens as a rule can be preserved intact, but if infiltrated with growth they should of course be removed. The remaining fascial connections of the bladder are severed, and it is finally detached by a horizontal incision through the prostate which is much the most difficult part of the operation. In females the urethra can be clamped, and the bladder removed much easier than in the male. Haemostasis is attended to and a drainage tube left in the cavity for a few days, and the abdominal wall closed.

PERURETHRAL OPERATIONS

(1) Small calculi and foreign bodies can often be removed from the cavity of the bladder through the operating cysto-urethroscope by one accustomed to its use.

(2) The treatment of papillomata by means of the diathermic current is in most cases easily carried out and is comparatively free from risk.

Small growths can be dealt with, after local anaesthetization of the urethra only, by means of a small electrode passed through the channel of an ordinary catheterizing cystoscope. Larger growths receive greater benefit from a heavier electrode, which may necessitate the use of an operating cystoscope and spinal or general anaesthesia.

Technique. The urethra having been anaesthetized, the patient is placed on the cystoscopic table, care being taken to see that he is suitably insulated. This is best effected by placing one or two rubber macintoshes or sorbo cushions between himself and the table. The indifferent electrode consisting of a flat metal sheet enclosed in several thicknesses of lint soaked in hypertonic saline is placed on the suprapubic region or under the buttocks. The catheterizing cystoscope is introduced and the growth inspected after lavage of the bladder with sterile water. The use of antiseptic bladder washes tends to make the liquid a conductor of electricity and thereby lessens the concentration of current at the positive electrode, on which ground they are not recommended when diathermy is to take place.

The positive electrode, having been passed through the catheterizing channel, appears in the visual field and is pushed on towards the growth. The Albarran lever may be actuated to bring the electrode into contact with the papilloma. The current is then turned on by means of the foot switch, and different areas of the growth treated for a few seconds at a time. These areas rapidly blanch until the whole or a considerable part of the tumour appears white and shrivelled as a result. Portions of the villi may become detached, or may adhere to the electrode. Small bubbles of hydrogen make their appearance at the positive pole during the passage of the current, which may be applied without much fear to growths on the base or lateral aspects of the bladder; but when these are situated on the upper aspect in close proximity to the peritoneal covering, caution should be maintained to prevent a possibility of perforation and subsequent peritonitis.

Provided the growth alone is treated the patient will complain of nothing beyond a gentle tingling, but if the normal mucous membrane inadvertently receives attention from the electrode a sharp pricking sensation—similar to the sting of a wasp—is felt.

Several sittings may be necessary to effect complete removal of a growth, and repeated cystoscopic examinations will be called for at later dates to determine the possibility of recurrence.

Patients vary greatly in their tolerance of this treatment, which should not exceed a duration of more than a minute or two at the first sitting.

(3) **Litholapaxy.** This operation is the method of choice amongst urological surgeons, and should be employed wherever possible. A cystoscopic lithotrite, cannulae and evacuator are necessary. The armamentarium designed by the late Canny Ryall is excellent for this purpose.

Technique. A preliminary X-ray and cystoscopy having been carried out, the size, shape and probable hardness of the stone will have been determined. A spinal anaesthetic is usually advisable, although in tolerant patients anaesthetization of the urethra alone may be sufficient. If the meatus is small a meatotomy will be called for. The cystoscopic lithotrite is introduced into the bladder which is distended with fluid to the limits of tolerance, the stone inspected, and grasped between its jaws. The cystoscope is partially withdrawn along its channel to protect it during crushing, and after depressing the handle to raise the stone from the bladder base it is steadily compressed by turning the screw until fracture results. The cystoscope is pushed along the channel and the resultant particles of the stone crushed until a satisfactory smallness is attained. The instrument is withdrawn and a cystoscopic cannula introduced. The evacuating bulb having been filled with fluid is then attached and the bladder contents subjected to alternate compression and suction until particles of stone cease to appear in the glass container. Lastly the cystoscope is introduced through the cannula, and the bladder inspected to note if any particles of stone are left behind—further suction by the evacuator being necessary if this is found to be the case. Emptying the bladder and removal of the cannula complete the operation.

Chapter IX

GENITO-URINARY TUBERCULOSIS

Genito-urinary tuberculosis may commence in kidney, prostate, testis, vesicula seminalis, or, rarely, Fallopian tube. Notwithstanding in whichever of these organs the "primary" focus is situated, the initial signs and symptoms are almost invariably first evidenced in the bladder, which sooner or later becomes secondarily attacked by the tubercle bacillus. For this reason it has been deemed advisable to consider tuberculosis of the genito-urinary tract as a whole in a separate and single chapter (Fig. 24).

The word "primary" is used in the narrow sense as referring to the first focus in this system, in spite of the fact that other foci in lungs, glands or bone may have been present for many years.

Formerly, as the result of animal experiments, it was held that renal tuberculosis might result from a "primary" focus in the bladder ascending the ureter. Clinically this has never been substantiated, and it is a good working principle to consider any vesical tuberculous lesion as invariably secondary to a focus situated elsewhere in the genito-urinary system—most commonly the kidney (95 per cent.).

RENAL TUBERCULOSIS

This is a blood-borne infection, most frequent between the ages of 20 and 40. It occurs slightly more often in females than males. Although commonly stated to be unilateral in the early stages, becoming bilateral later, there is some reason to doubt this assertion.

Clinically the signs are unilateral in the early stages, but a small and latent focus may be present in the other kidney

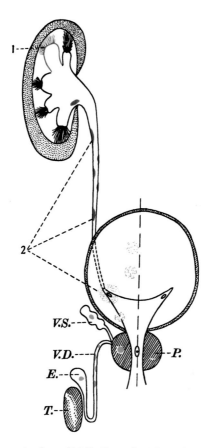

Fig. 24. Diagram to show distribution of genito-urinary tuberculosis. Urinary tuberculosis (red). Primary focus in kidney 1. Secondary foci in ureter and circumureteric region of bladder. 2. Genital tuberculosis (green). Primary foci in epididymis, prostate, and vesicula seminalis. Secondary foci in vas deferens, and bladder (not necessarily circumureteric in position). *V.S.* Vesicula seminalis. *V.D.* Vas deferens. *E.* Epididymis. *T.* Testicle. *P.* Prostate.

which becomes manifest if the progress of the disease is not arrested. Superimposed infection with the *B. coli* or other organism is common in the advanced stages.

Pathology:

Kidney. (1) A tuberculous pyonephrosis, which differs only in its aetiology from any other pyonephrosis.

(2) Tuberculous ulceration. This form generally commences at the base of a pyramid, first as an inflamed area to be followed later by patches of caseation and eventual destruction until large cavities in the kidney parenchyma are formed.

Ureter. In both forms sooner or later the ureter becomes affected, patches of ulceration appear on the mucosa, its wall is densely thickened and infiltrated, and by its retraction its lower orifice may be pulled upwards from the bladder with the resultant formation of a trumpet-shaped opening. In other cases where the ureter is no longer capable of contraction its lower end may be widely open, circular, and resembling the cavity of a "golf hole".

Bladder. The pathology of tuberculous cystitis differs to some extent with the seat of the primary lesion. Small grey or yellowish tubercles make their appearance deep to the mucous membrane and, on breaking down, give rise to a small erosion. The coalescence of these erosions forms ulcers similar to tuberculous ulceration in other parts of the body. The base is a pale pink, and the edges undermined.

If the primary focus is situated in the kidney, tubercle bacilli *may* reach the bladder in the urinary stream through the ureter, or, as is more generally held (without, it must be admitted, very conclusive proof), via the periureteric lymphatic plexus. Whichever route is taken by these bacilli, the first sign of their arrival in the bladder will become manifest in the neighbourhood of the ureteric orifice on the affected side.

When the primary focus is localized in the prostate, vesiculae, or epididymis, the pathological changes taking place in the bladder are not so closely related to the ureteric opening, though they are usually situated in close proximity to the trigone.

In untreated cases ulceration progresses until the deeper tissues of the bladder are invaded, with an increase in pain and a loss of elasticity in the bladder wall.

Signs and Symptoms. The earliest signs and symptoms of urinary tuberculosis are generally manifest in the bladder. Their great importance lies in the fact that they represent the outward and visible manifestations of a primary focus situated elsewhere. They may be conveniently grouped under the headings—early, intermediate, and late.

Early. The spontaneous appearance of frequency and polyuria in a young individual with an acid urine should always raise the suspicion of a tuberculous lesion. The polyuria may be unilateral, and then indicates the site of the lesion. In this stage the polyuria probably denotes an attempt on the part of the kidney to rid itself of noxious products by copious watery "flushings" and a resultant frequency.

Intermediate. In the second stage, frequency becomes more marked owing to tuberculous infection at the lower end of the ureter and bladder. Haematuria may occur either from kidney or bladder sources and is extremely variable in amount. About this time pyuria makes its appearance, and tubercle bacilli may be found in the urine. Definite changes take place in the mucous membrane of the bladder with the production of hyperaemic, oedematous, or ulcerated areas, visible on cystoscopy, and in close proximity to the infected ureter. With the development of ulceration in the bladder, painful micturition becomes a marked symptom. Pain in the kidney is not prominent, but this organ may be tender on palpation and a dull ache is not uncommon.

Late. In the advanced stages extensive ulceration of the bladder occurs, and owing to the infiltration of its walls it becomes indistensible—holding only a few drachms of urine. Frequency is intense and often intolerable, and micturition may occur at 15-min. intervals, associated with a severity of pain which renders the patient's life a misery. Pyuria is profuse, and mixed infections common. The affected kidney is sometimes tender and, when of the pyonephrotic type, enlarged. Increase in the size of the kidney, however, is no guide to the side of the disease, as the unaffected kidney is not uncommonly enlarged as a compensating mechanism to the destroyed organ, and may be tender although devoid of tubercular lesions. A tender, palpable, ureter is sometimes found, and its lower end may be palpable as a hard cord *per vaginam* or *per rectum*. Untreated, the course is progressive. Pain, frequency, haematuria and pyuria increase. The second kidney becomes infected in a vast majority of cases, the patient dying from uraemia, exhaustion or superimposed septic infection.

Investigation. In well-marked cases of tuberculous cystitis with pain, frequency and pyuria in which tubercle bacilli have been found, the identification of the primary focus may not be difficult. In the early cases, however, before tubercle bacilli have been found in the urine, considerable difficulty may be experienced in deciding firstly the nature of the cystitis, and secondly the organ primarily responsible for it.

The clinical examination should be directed towards the condition of the kidneys, prostate, testes, vesiculae seminales, and the Fallopian tubes. A rectal examination may reveal tender and swollen nodules in prostate or vesiculae, whilst scrotal palpation may show an enlarged epididymis or an irregularly "beaded" vas deferens. A vaginal examination may bring to light a diseased Fallopian tube.

Radiology will prove or exclude the presence of vesical calculi, and the condition of a tuberculous kidney is occasionally demonstrated on the X-ray film. Excretion urography sometimes proves of great value in demonstrating cavitation of the kidney, and abnormal extensions of the renal pelvis. Furthermore it gives some indication of the functional capacity of the kidneys in relation to one another.

In practically every case, however, cystoscopy will be necessary, and if there is much frequency and pain it is better to carry this out under a spinal or general anaesthetic rather than attempt the dilatation of an intolerant bladder after local anaesthetization of the urethra alone. In the earliest stages of **renal** tuberculosis during the period of unilaterality, the ureteric orifice of the affected side and its immediate surroundings may be slightly swollen and hyperaemic. Later, small vesicles or tubercles may become apparent, or a loss of epithelium amounting to ulceration may occur. The mucous membrane appears thicker and more rigid than normal, and a bullous oedema may occur at the trigone. The urinary efflux is often difficult to see, although urine may be ejected almost continuously and, at any rate in the early stages, the measure of urine from the affected kidney is nearly always much in excess of that of the normal side.

As the disease progresses with infiltration and retraction of the ureter, changes in the shape of the ureteric orifice become apparent. The opening becomes rigid, and trumpet-shaped, or even "golf hole" in contour, signifying a function-less kidney. The intravesical portion of the ureter may become more obvious as a thickened ridge. Ulceration may be well marked, and in some cases granulations may be present.

In tuberculosis of the genital organs with secondary extension to the bladder, ureteric changes will be absent, and the diagnosis will rest on the presence of characteristic ulceration and tubercle bacilli in the pus—if necessary backed up by ureteric catheterization revealing normal urine from either ureter.

Treatment. No local treatment of the bladder is of any avail, and should not be instigated. Removal of the primary cause, if that is possible, should be carried out, after which in most cases the tuberculous condition of the bladder will rapidly subside. This is effected by means of a nephrectomy when the focus is in the kidney; when situated in testis or vesicula seminalis these must be removed.

The administration of urinary antiseptics may prevent or modify a superimposed infection with other organisms, but has no effect on the tubercle bacillus.

If the primary focus cannot be removed (e.g. bilateral renal lesions), or if after removal cystitis shows no signs of improvement, and severe pain and intense frequency is present, particularly if the bladder is contracted (systolic bladder), transplantation of the ureters (or remaining ureter) into the sigmoid should be carried out. The results of this operation are excellent when judged by the relief afforded to the patient, who soon learns to hold his or her urine in the rectum for 3 or 4 hours during the day, and 6 or 8 at night.

TUBERCULOSIS OF PROSTATE

Tuberculosis of the prostate is most commonly seen in young adults, and is frequently associated with tuberculous disease of kidney, bladder, vesicula and testis. A previous gonorrhoea is generally admitted. The symptoms are those of a prostatitis, and rectal examination reveals a tender and nodular gland. Treatment is unsatisfactory. In a minority of cases prostatectomy is possible. Abscesses and fistulae call for curettage and excision.

TUBERCULOSIS OF VESICULAE SEMINALES

Tuberculosis of vesiculae seminales is usually associated with tuberculous disease of testis or prostate. Pain and weight in the perineum are occasionally present, and the vesicula feels hard and nodular in the early stages, or soft and fluctuating in the later. Treatment consists in its removal by the perineal route in the primary condition, or in association with orchidectomy if the testis is diseased as well.

TUBERCULOSIS OF TESTIS AND VAS DEFERENS

In the early stages this takes the form of an epididymo-orchitis, and may be acute or chronic. The acute condition might be confused with gonorrhoea but for the absence of a discharge. In the chronic form a nodule appears in the epididymis. Later the skin of the scrotum becomes adherent to the back of the testis, and abscesses form which may discharge with the formation of a sinus. The vas may be normal, or enlarged and hard like a slate pencil. In other cases nodules appear on it (beaded vas). Other foci in vesiculae or prostate are commonly found. A secondary hydrocele is sometimes present.

Treatment. Orchidectomy is the operation of choice although epididymectomy is occasionally justifiable.

TUBERCULOSIS OF THE FEMALE GENERATIVE ORGANS

For details see works on Gynaecology.

Chapter X

THE URETHRA

ANATOMY

The male urethra is divided by anatomists into three main parts:

    (1) Prostatic.
    (2) Membraneous.
    (3) Bulbous (*a*) perineal,
               (*b*) penile.

Clinically, the urethra is more conveniently divided into anterior and posterior parts, the dividing line being the triangular ligaments (urogenital trigone) with their contained sphincter.

The prostatic urethra will vary in length with the size of the prostate, but is normally about an inch long. Its direction is downwards and slightly forwards, and on its posterior wall is a well-marked eminence, the verumontanum (Crista Galli, Colliculus), on which open the common ejaculatory ducts, while the orifices of the prostatic ducts open into the lateral bays on either side of it. This prominence gives to the prostatic urethra a horseshoe-shaped lumen. It is an exquisitely sensitive structure and has been described as the "trigger area" of ejaculation and urination. The internal urinary meatus, normally closed by circular muscle fibres acting as a sphincter, has the appearance in miniature of the anal orifice.

The membraneous urethra—$\frac{1}{2}$ in. in length, situated between the two layers of the triangular ligaments (urogenital trigone), and surrounded by the well-marked sphincter urethrae membranaceae muscle—is the narrowest part of the urethral lumen with the exception of the external urinary meatus, and is directed downwards and forwards.

The bulbous urethra lies inside the corpus spongiosum, and runs forwards and very slightly upwards to the under surface of the symphysis pubis, from which point it turns downwards into the penis and is subdivided into a perineal and penile portion. The perineal part lies between Colles fascia and the under surface of the lower layer of the triangular ligament in the perineum, and receives the openings of the ducts of Cowper's glands. Its lumen, together with that of the penile urethra—exclusive of the terminal 1 in.—is a horizontal oval. It is about 3 in. long.

The penile urethra—a continuation of the perineal part of the bulbous urethra—lies distal to the symphysis in the penis, and will vary in extent with the length of that organ. In the glans penis the lumen is fusiform with a well-marked diverticulum on its dorsal wall (the lacuna magna), and in this region it is sometimes referred to as the fossa navicularis. It opens to the exterior by a vertical slit, the external urinary meatus—the narrowest part of the urethral lumen. Into both the perineal and penile parts of the bulbous urethra open numerous glands (of Littré). Thus, the male urethra with a flaccid penis makes an ∽-shaped curve, descending from the bladder, ascending to the symphysis, and running downwards and forwards in the penis. This curve will be modified by the introduction *per urethram* of certain instruments. Only with a rubber catheter does this canal retain its normal contour. When a well-curved metal prostatic catheter is used, a c-shaped canal will result, while the insertion into the bladder of urethroscope and cystoscope renders the urethral canal straight from external to internal orifices.

The lymphatic vessels of the urethra discharge their lymph into the inguinal, external and internal iliac lymph glands.

The female urethra is $1\frac{1}{2}$ in. long and is closely bound up with the anterior wall of the vagina. The external urinary meatus varies greatly in position in different individuals. Little notice of this extreme variation appears to have been taken by anatomists. The urethra is surrounded close to the bladder by Skene's tubules, which appear to be the female counterpart of the prostate in the male.

DEFORMITIES

Certain congenital deformities of the urethra not uncommonly occur.

(1) Very rarely, an imperforate or septate urethra—usually associated with a patent urachus or opening into the rectum —has been described. Still more rarely these safety-valve openings may be absent.

(2) Hypospadias is a condition in which the floor of the urethra for a variable length has failed to develop, and the external urinary meatus may be situated at any point from under the surface of the glans to just in front of the anus.

Three types have been described.

(a) The opening is situated anywhere on the under surface of the glans (glandular hypospadias).

(b) The opening is situated anywhere between the corona glandis and the scrotum (penile hypospadias).

(c) The opening is situated in the perineum. It is nearly always associated with undescended testes, rudimentary penis, and closely resembles the appearance of the vulva. No vagina, however, is present (perineal hypospadias).

Treatment of Hypospadias. No surgical treatment is necessary as a rule in glandular hypospadias, unless it be the dilatation of a minute orifice. In the perineal type no treatment is practicable. In penile hypospadias various plastic operations have been devised, for details of which the student is referred to works on operative surgery. On the whole, operation is unsatisfactory, and a temporary suprapubic cystotomy for the purpose of diverting the urine is nearly always necessary. In view of the otherwise normal development of these individuals and the distressing results of a penile hypospadias, treatment is justified as long as the length of its duration and the not infrequent failures and difficulties are explained to the parents.

(3) The condition of epispadias is the reverse of hypospadias, the external urinary meatus opening anywhere along the dorsum of the penis. Its development is difficult to explain and has been thought to be due to one of two causes:

(a) Either a deficiency in the dorsal wall of the urethra, or

(b) Rotation through 180° of a hypospadias.

It is always associated with a minute penis, and in many cases with undescended testes, unjoined symphysis pubis, and ectopia vesicae.

Treatment of Epispadias. In partial conditions of this deformity with urinary control, plastic operations, although difficult, are justifiable. Where possible they should be carried out when the child is 3 or 4 years old. Where epispadias is associated with ectopia vesicae, or non-control of micturition, ureteric transplantation into the sigmoid should be performed.

RUPTURE OF THE URETHRA

Rupture of the urethra is usually caused by external violence applied to the perineum, e.g. kicks, falling astride a gate, or in conjunction with a fractured pelvis. It may be complete or partial.

The patient complains of severe pain with local bruising and tenderness, and if the rupture be in the anterior urethra, blood will escape from the external meatus independent of micturition. There may be a strong desire to pass water, but if possible the patient must be dissuaded from this action. If, however, urination has been attempted—with perhaps partial success—extravasation will have resulted and will give rise to signs which vary with the site of the rupture. The usual sites of rupture are:

(1) Perineal.

(2) Intrapelvic.

The first is much the commoner; the second is usually associated with fracture of the pelvis.

A ruptured urethra may be diagnosed when local pain, urethral haemorrhage, perineal haematoma and retention of urine occur, but unfortunately the severity and degree of the rupture cannot be determined from these signs.

Investigation and Treatment. Investigation and treatment should proceed hand in hand, the writer being of opinion that casual instrumentation and catheterization are strongly to be deprecated.

The patient should be anaesthetized by general or spinal anaesthesia, and, with full precautions and gentleness, the condition of the urethra inspected with the irrigating urethroscope. In cases of partial rupture it is probably justifiable to pass a catheter into the bladder, if this can be easily effected. It may be left *in situ* for 24 hours, after which it should be removed. A careful watch should be kept on the perineum, and any sign of suppuration dealt with by immediate incision.

In cases of complete rupture immediate operation should be proceeded with. The great difficulty in exposing the vesical end of the divided urethra is well known, and many varied manœuvres have been suggested for rendering it apparent.

If the two ends of the divided urethra are not rapidly exposed through the perineal incision, no time should be wasted but a suprapubic cystotomy should be performed and retrograde catheterization via the prostatic urethra carried out. The most useful instruments for this manœuvre are a Lister's sound, a red rubber catheter, or a urethral guide, which can be made to appear at the perineal opening, thus defining the vesical end of the urethra. The distal severed end can be made prominent by a sound passed from the external urinary meatus. Some authorities recommend that cystotomy and retrograde catheterization should be the first step in the treatment of every case before searching the perineum for the divided urethral ends, as they hold that transferring the patient from the lithotomy to the recumbent position and back again requires extra manipulation, and encourages sepsis.

Several methods have been adopted in the past for approximating and fixing the divided urethral ends. Guyon, the pioneer, and numerous followers have sutured the divided urethra end to end round an indwelling catheter. Rutherford, of Glasgow, after preliminary suprapubic cystotomy and identification of the severed ends of the urethra, introduced a rubber catheter along the whole length of the urethra into the bladder but made no attempt to suture the divided ends, leaving suprapubic and perineal wounds open, obtaining excellent results thereby.

Where extravasation of urine or much sepsis is present suture of the urethra is impossible, and the introduction of a urethral catheter along the whole length of the urethra is probably unnecessary, a free exposure with approximation of the two parts of the urethra being all that is required— anything of the nature of a foreign body being excluded, e.g. sutures and catheter. When these complications are absent, an excellent result may be obtained by suture of the dorsal wall of the urethra—two or three stitches are sufficient—and leaving a catheter *in situ* between the **perineal** wound and the bladder only. The suprapubic opening in the bladder, in this case, may be closed if a drain is left down to it, or sewn up tightly round a rubber tube which may be removed after 4 or 5 days.

If the bladder is drained, as in the latter alternative, no catheter need be left in the vesical part of the urethra, but the foot of the bed should be raised to assist drainage of urine by the suprapubic tube.

Whichever method is adopted, the perineal wound is left open and lightly packed with gauze which has been soaked in some mild antiseptic. Attention is directed to rendering this wound as free from sepsis as possible by frequent irrigation with hydrogen peroxide or eusol. A Canny Ryall syringe will be found admirable for this procedure.

A metal sound of medium dimension should be passed about the tenth day, and repeated at intervals of 3 or 4 days until the perineal wound is healed.

Later, urethroscopic examination should take place at monthly intervals—for the first few months—to guard against contracture: still later, the occasional passage of a large-sized metal sound (or better, a Kollmann's dilator) can be instituted at increasingly longer intervals.

Intrapelvic rupture of the urethra most commonly occurs in conjunction with a fractured pelvis, and usually at the point where prostatic and membraneous urethrae join. The condition is more serious than perineal rupture, and extravasation of urine takes place early, giving rise to a tender swelling in the hypogastric region often mistaken for a distended bladder (cf. Figs. 25, 26). Urethroscopy, under a general or spinal anaesthetic, may yield valuable information. More commonly an extraperitoneal rupture of the bladder will be diagnosed and operation undertaken for this. At exploration, the bladder will be found intact—probably containing some urine—while blood-stained and extravasated urine is present below, in front, and at the sides of the bladder. Owing to the rupture of the pubo-prostatic ligaments, the neck of the bladder is dislocated backwards, and unless steps are taken in the first few days to rectify this, before fixation in this abnormal position occurs, reconstruction of the urethra is most unlikely (Fig. 26). Immediate treatment consists in the

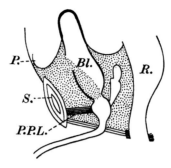

Fig. 25. Diagram to show extraperitoneal rupture of bladder with urinary extravasation. [Pubo-prostatic ligaments and urethra intact. Urine shown by dots.] *Bl.*, Bladder. *P.*, Peritoneum. *P.P.L.*, Pubo-prostatic ligaments. *R.*, Rectum. *S.*, Symphysis.

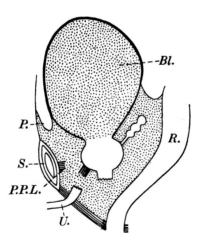

Fig. 26. Diagram to show intrapelvic rupture of urethra with urinary extravasation. [Pubo-prostatic ligaments and urethra ruptured, bladder intact but neck dislocated backwards. Urine shown by dots.] *Bl.*, Bladder *P.*, Peritoneum. *P.P.L.*, Pubo-prostatic ligaments. *R.*, Rectum. *S.*, Symphysis. *U.*, Urethra.

drainage of the extravasated urine and the performance of a suprapubic cystotomy. When the bladder is open, a Lister's sound can be passed in a retrograde manner through the prostatic urethra and made to project into the perineum from inside the bulbous urethra, where it can be exposed by an incision in this region. A catheter attached to the end of this sound can be pulled up into the bladder and retained for 10 days. This catheter will prevent fixation of the bladder neck in the backwardly dislocated position, and once introduced the posterior end of the urethra is under control. On its withdrawal, careful and painstaking instrumentation will allow the perineal wound to heal and normal reunion of the divided urethra to take place.

EXTRAVASATION OF URINE

"Extravasation of urine" is far less common than formerly. As has been mentioned, when urine is extravasated from the prostatic urethra or from extraperitoneal rupture of the bladder it diffuses into the perivesical tissues of the pelvis.

Extravasation from the membraneous urethra alone has never been described. Theoretically, it should remain between the two layers of the triangular ligaments, with the possibility of a track along the dorsal vein of the penis along the upper surface of that organ.

Extravasation from the bulbous urethra is limited by the attachments of the fascia of Colles when this is intact. It will extend backwards to the anus, laterally to the junction between thigh and perineum, forwards to the integuments of scrotum and penis, and upwards along the anterior abdominal wall for a variable distance. Though uncommon apart from rupture of the urethra, it can occur in cases of periurethral suppuration, and its possibility should be borne in mind in any case presenting a swollen, oedematous, or blackish penis, scrotum and perineum. The treatment consists in evacuating the extravasated urine by suitably planned incisions at the earliest possible moment.

FOREIGN BODIES AND CALCULUS
FOREIGN BODIES

Foreign bodies introduced into the urethra are not very unusual—slate pencils and hairpins being the most common. If recently introduced they can usually be extracted by the aid of the urethroscope and suitable forceps. If left *in situ* for a few days they give rise to a discharge which may be confused with gonorrhoea, unless a reliable history of their introduction is obtained. In old-standing cases ulceration may take place, and the foreign body, together with blood, pus and urine, pass to the exterior. A urinary fistula may form, or a stricture develop at the site of ulceration.

CALCULUS

Calculi situated in the urethra are nearly always secondary to foci elsewhere; e.g. small renal or ureteric calculi, previously passed into the bladder, may, by deposit on their surface, become too great to pass through the whole length of the urethra, or may be arrested at the site of a stricture. Calculi derived from the prostate may behave in a similar manner. They give rise to a diminished, or suddenly arrested stream. Haematuria and pyuria may occur, and the calculus can usually be felt *per rectum*, or in the perineum and penis. Sometimes they can be seen at the external urinary orifice. If not visible to the naked eye a urethroscope will localize them, and as a rule they can be dislodged and extracted *per urethram* by spoon, or a combination of urethroscopic forceps and digital manœuvres carried out under local anaesthesia.

STRICTURE OF THE URETHRA

Stricture, or narrowing of the urethra, may be due to trauma (e.g. rupture), or result from previous inflammation and ulceration—most commonly gonorrhoeal in nature—with the consequent sclerosis of subepithelial tissues which invades the surrounding parts, and by its contracture diminishes or occludes the urethral calibre.

Many names are in use to describe different types of stricture (e.g. resilient or elastic, cartilaginous, impassable), but fundamentally this condition results from narrowing of the urethral canal by fibrosis at one or more points. Formerly, chiefly owing to the casual or inefficient treatment of gonorrhoea, stricture of the urethra was very common between the ages of 25 and 55. Nowadays, however, it is far less often met with, for the reason previously mentioned.

Clinical History. A young or middle-aged man giving a past history of gonorrhoea or urethral injury, complaining of difficulty in micturition with a small stream, together with a normal-sized prostate, is almost certainly the victim of urethral stricture. Frequency is sometimes present, and retention may occur. In addition, stricture may be complicated by septic conditions of any part of the urinary tract, or even its neighbourhood, e.g. epididymitis and periurethritis. Signs of back pressure on bladder, ureter and kidney may be manifest with consequent impairment of their function.

Investigation. The investigation of a stricture, after due attention has been given to the history, should be commenced by the administration of the local anaesthetic described in chapter II. This should be followed, in most cases, by a urethroscopy when the face of the stricture can be inspected and any false passages noted.

If a urethroscope is not available, the position and size of the stricture can be estimated by passing gum-elastic bougies of diminishing size until one can be found to traverse the stricture—the commencing bougie being of at least size No. 10 E. If no bougie can be made to pass, a gum-elastic guide to which a following sound or bougie can be attached can often be introduced. These flexible guides (filiform), which are made of gum elastic—sometimes surrounding a wire—possess a screw socket at one end into which

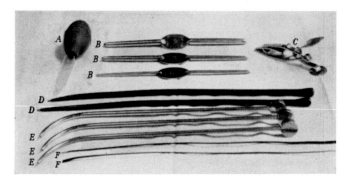

Fig. 27. Urethral instruments. *A*, Canny Ryall syringe. *B, B, B*, Meatal dilators. *C*, Penile clamp. *D, D*, Gum-elastic followers. *E, E, E*, Curved metal followers. *F, F*, Flexible guides with screw socket.

graduated followers can be screwed and made to follow the track of the guide into the bladder. The guide can often be made to enter the narrow mouth of the stricture by bending the point to an angle of 120°, and by a combination of advancement, rotation and retraction, the elusive opening may be found.

The writer is of opinion that small metal sounds of size 10/14 (Clutton's) or less calibre should not be employed in the investigation of stricture, unless made to screw into a preliminary guide.

Treatment. Stricture, *per se*, would have little or no ill-effects on a patient were it not for the complications it brings in its train. In the past, attention was directed to the prevention or relief of acute urinary obstruction only, to which end means were taken to render the stricture barely permeable, without consideration of the evils of back pressure on renal function. Nowadays, every attempt is made to prevent not only acute retention but the more distant complications of chronic retention, infection, back pressure and renal failure,

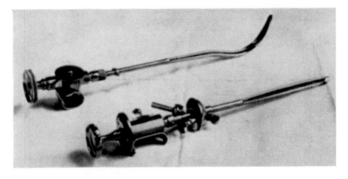

Fig. 28. Kollmann's dilators, curved and straight.

by increasing the narrowed urethral lumen to normal, or even greater, dimensions. This may be carried out by gradual dilatation or, in some cases, by cutting operations, e.g. internal urethrotomy. In most cases dilatation is the method of choice and, except in the presence of gross urethral sepsis or impassable stricture, is nearly always employed.

Bougies of increasing size are passed through the stricture under local anaesthesia. When a bougie of size 12 can be successfully passed, Clutton's or Lister's sounds may be substituted, or better the straight—and later curved—expanding dilators of Kollmann (Fig. 28). The expansion of these instruments is indicated on a dial, and dilatation of the stricture should be proceeded with until the curved instrument can be expanded to size 35 or 40 without discomfort to the patient.

Effective local anaesthetization and numerous sittings are essential, dilatation being carried out very gradually at intervals of a week or 10 days until full dilatation is reached.

It is inadvisable to pass more than two instruments through the stricture at a sitting—the larger size to remain *in situ* for 20 min. When the Kollmann's dilator is used it can be screwed open to the dial mark 25 without difficulty, after which point each further degree will encounter more resistance. Three to five additional degrees are ample for a sitting. The full limit of dilatation of the stricture will vary with the size of the urethra, and will lie between Nos. 35 and 45 on the dial of the curved Kollmann's dilator. When this limit is reached, several sittings of full dilatation lasting over a period of 2 or 3 months will be necessary.

The time necessary to effect a "cure" varies, of course, with the severity of the stricture, but will seldom be less than several months, and can rarely be effective unless the increasing dilatation can be carried out painlessly. It cannot be too strongly emphasized that all those cases which are being pronounced "cured" should at least be subjected to a urethroscopic review for a year or two after the cessation of active treatment, when a recurrent contraction of the stricture can be immediately noted and countered. If this is not feasible, some kind of large metal instrument should be passed once or twice a year as a protection against recontraction.

In the presence of sepsis in and around the urethra, dilatation of the stricture should, as far as possible, be delayed until the sepsis has been treated.

Certain strictures—for example those in which dilatation is unsatisfactory either by reason of the difficulty in performing it or the elastic nature of the stricture—are unsuitable for dilatation by bougies, and the operation of internal urethrotomy may be called for.

Opinions differ greatly as to the indications for this operation, which at any rate is performed far less frequently than in days gone by. It consists in passing a guide, to which can be attached an instrument with a guarded blade, through the stricture, which can be made to sever the fibrous tissue— care being taken to keep the blade in midline between the two corpora cavernosa. Its chief danger is the occurrence of haemorrhage, and on its withdrawal a catheter should always be tied into the bladder for 4 days, after which dilatation by means of bougies and Kollmann's dilators should be proceeded with. In the hands of experts it gives excellent results with a low mortality.

External urethrotomy, as a method of treating uncomplicated stricture, is nowadays but rarely called for, and is usually reserved for impassable strictures after a preliminary drainage of the bladder.

Excision of the stricture is sometimes practised with good results, if the stricture is single and its extent not too great. As in the treatment of ruptured urethra, the dorsal wall only of this channel should be sutured and a catheter introduced through the opening in the perineal urethra into the bladder. The operation, however, is difficult and of considerable magnitude, and should not be lightly undertaken until the full extent of its possibilities have been considered.

Where the patient's general condition is poor, as for instance if renal function is impaired as evidenced by high blood urea, thirst, "parrot tongue", or low urea concentration, it may be necessary to perform a preliminary cystotomy. This is more likely to be called for as a first stage in the subsequent treatment of stricture by the cutting operations, when it should not be unduly withheld. It should be borne in mind that chronic urinary back pressure may be brought about as easily by stricture as by the enlarged prostate, for which the two-stage operation is accepted as a common necessity even by the lay public.

When stricture is complicated by acute retention of urine other methods may be called for, as the first essential is the relief of stress on the over-full bladder.

If a catheter can be passed the urine can be withdrawn and dilatation proceeded with at once, or better still the catheter may be left *in situ* and dilatation commenced the next day.

If a catheter cannot be passed, it may be possible to traverse the stricture with a flexible guide to which a following catheter can be screwed, and the bladder emptied of its contents. If there has been great difficulty in passing the filiform guide into the bladder, it should be retained in the urethra for 24 hours, when dilatation can be continued without having to submit to prolonged manipulation in order to find anew the elusive orifice of the stricture. Urine will pass beside it, and its presence in the stricture will probably result in slight increase in diameter at this region. If in spite of all a catheter cannot be made to enter the bladder, one of two methods should be adopted:

(a) The bladder contents may be emptied by suprapubic puncture with trocar and cannula, after which with the lessening of strictural spasm it may be possible to pass, and tie in, a catheter, or guide;

or (b) Suprapubic cystotomy may be performed, when it will usually be found possible to manœuvre a catheter through the stricture into the bladder. Retrograde catheterization may be necessary to effect this.

If in spite of suprapubic cystotomy no instrument can be made to pass the stricture at the first attempt, acute retention

will have been relieved, and at a later date it may be comparatively easy to traverse the stricture. It should not be
forgotten that great help can often be derived from urethroscopy, for example when the ureteric catheter can be made
to enter the diminutive mouth of the stricture under the
guidance of the eye and pushed on from there into the
bladder.

URETHRITIS

The urethra is very resistant to micro-organisms descending
from above, but is easily infected from the external meatus
either by organisms introduced with unclean instruments, or
by the gonococcus at coitus. It is probable that though the
gonococcus can traverse a normal mucous membrane and
give rise to a purulent urethritis, other organisms can only
infect the urethra when a greater or lesser degree of trauma
is present—as witnessed by the frequent urethral discharge
after clumsy instrumentation, particularly if false passages
have been formed.

For the diagnosis, complications, and treatment of gonorrhoeal urethritis the reader is referred to works on venereal
disease.

Other types of urethritis, though rare, occur most commonly from the effects of the *B. coli*, and a thin watery discharge (in contrast to the thick creamy pus of gonorrhoea) is
present. Extension to testis and epididymis is not uncommon, and whenever a urethral discharge other than
gonorrhoeal is found, the possibility of a retained foreign
body should be considered.

Microscopic investigation of the pus should be one's first
care. Instrumentation of a urethra acutely infected with
gonorrhoea is strongly contraindicated, even if retention has
supervened. In these cases, suprapubic aspiration is safer
than catheterization. Once gonorrhoea has been excluded

a routine examination can be carried out, and treatment commenced.

The treatment consists of copious fluids by mouth, of which the most useful are barley water, lemonade and cherry-stalk tea. This latter is not so well known as it merits in England, but is of definite value both as a diuretic and a mild urinary antiseptic. Alkalis, hyoscyamus, and acriflavine gr. ½ by mouth are often useful adjuncts. Gentle irrigation of the urethra with potassium permanganate or oxycyanide of mercury is useful. Alcohol and sexual activity should be avoided.

PERIURETHRITIS

(Abscess and Fistula)

Periurethritis may take the form of a hard inflammatory swelling surrounding the perineal urethra, in which multiple small abscesses are found. It results from infection extending from the confines of the urethra to its neighbourhood, from ulceration behind a stricture, round a foreign body or false passage. In more acute cases well-marked suppuration may occur, and a large abscess may form. Signs of local inflammation become evident and pain may be a marked feature. When diagnosed it should be incised. Hot baths are useful both before and after operation. A foreign body may be extruded with the pus, but when a stricture is present its treatment must be delayed until the signs of acute inflammation have subsided.

Urinary fistulae may occur in any part of the urinary tract. When connected with the urethra their external opening is in the perineum or penis. They often result from rupture, or imperfect drainage, of a periurethral abscess, or occur proximal to a stricture. Treatment consists in combating sepsis by free incision or excision of the track and dilatation of any stricture that may exist.

Chapter XI

THE PROSTATE

ANATOMY

The prostate resembles a horse-chestnut in shape and size. Situated at the neck of the bladder it surrounds the prostatic urethra, and consists of the following parts:

(1) A part anterior to the urethra in which glandular tissue is scanty, and fibro-muscular tissue predominant—the anterior lobe or commissure. Pathological enlargement of this lobe is rare.

(2) Two lateral lobes situated postero-lateral to the urethra in which glandular tissue predominates.

(3) A small "middle lobe" bounded in front by the urethra, above by the bladder, behind and below by the common ejaculatory ducts, and on either side by the lateral lobes. This part of the prostate, largely glandular in structure, normally projects slightly into the urethral orifice of the bladder to form the uvula vesicae. When pathologically enlarged it encroaches on the bladder lumen and occasionally acts as a ball valve to the urethra, with resultant urinary retention.

(4) A posterior lobe situated below the "middle lobe" in close relationship with the rectum.

The prostatic urethra is $1\frac{1}{4}$ in. long, and presents on its dorsal wall an elevation—the verumontanum—causing the lumen to be crescentic in shape. The organ is invested by connective tissue (visceral pelvic fascia), extensions of which pass forwards to the pubic bones as the pubo-prostatic ligaments. The prostatic ducts discharge their secretion into the urethra at the sides of the verumontanum.

Histologically the prostate consists of fifty or sixty separate glands, each opening by a separate duct into the urethra. Some of these lie in the posterior lobe, and have been referred to by continental writers as the "true prostatic glands". They form that part of the prostate which is palpable *per rectum.*

The remaining prostatic glands are periurethral in situation (anterior, lateral and "middle" lobes), and are partially separated from the posterior lobe by a layer of plain circular muscle fibre which surrounds the urethra and is continuous above with the bladder sphincter. The subcervical glands of Albarran form a small group which open into the posterior wall of the internal meatus above the "middle" lobe. "Prostatectomy" for benign enlargement of the gland probably consists only in a removal of the enlarged periurethral glands, leaving intact the posterior lobe—represented by a thin and atrophic layer of glandular tissue—while in the operation of Harris no attempt to remove the anterior commissure is made.

Examination of the prostate is carried out:

(a) *Per rectum.* The examining finger can detect enlargements of the posterior and lateral lobes, but not of "middle" or anterior lobes.

(b) By means of the cystoscope, whereby the "middle" and anterior lobes can be examined and intravesical projections of the lateral lobes noted. In many cases a well-marked prostatic "collar" can be found.

(c) By means of the urethroscope, where the encroachment of the prostate on the urethra and the condition of the internal urinary meatus can be determined.

PROSTATITIS

Acute and chronic forms of prostatitis occur. Gonorrhoea is the commonest cause in each case, although infection with other organisms—notably *B. coli communis*—occasionally occurs.

In the acute condition infection reaches the periurethral glandular part of the prostate, and intense inflammation progressing to suppuration or abscess formation results. Pain is present in the perineum and on micturition. Haematuria may occur. Tenderness, often very marked, is present in the rectum, and is made worse by the passage of a motion or by examination with the finger.

Chronic prostatitis is a common sequel of gonorrhoea. Infection of the ducts, with the formation of a fibrosis around them, results. "Threads" representing inspissated pus casts of the prostatic ducts appear in the urine, together with a persistent watery urethral discharge (gleet). Pain and weight in the perineum occur, and micturition may be painful. *Per rectum* the prostate is not very tender, and it can be emptied of discharge by finger pressure (massage).

A mild form of prostatitis, often associated with a *B. coli* bacilluria, is not very uncommon.

Clinically this occurs in young or middle-aged individuals of nervous temperament, and is characterized by frequency and urgency of micturition, pain at the end of the act, and is occasionally associated with the passage of a few drops of blood. Slight incontinence is not uncommon: a bacilluria is generally present, and *per rectum* the prostate feels swollen and rather tender.

Cystoscopically a trigonitis is seen, and not uncommonly the urethroscope reveals a sphincter vesicae which is atonic, and does not contract well on withdrawal of the instrument. This accounts for the patient's difficulty in holding his water, and is probably due to the swollen and oedematous prostate interfering with the normal functioning of the sphincteric mechanism of the bladder.

The condition is often associated with psychical changes in the patient—particularly impotence, which may be purely temporary in duration.

Treatment. Treatment of the acute condition takes the form of a veto on all sexual connection, alcoholic and other stimulating drinks, and the avoidance of all erotic surroundings and impulses. The bowels should be well regulated, and the patient confined to bed if possible. Fomentations to the perineum, or hip baths, together with copious bland fluids by the mouth are helpful. A mild urinary antiseptic (e.g. urotropine) is advisable, but it is doubtful if it has any effect on the cause of the disease. If an abscess forms, it generally ruptures spontaneously into urethra or rectum; or it may be necessary to open it through the rectum, or better still at its side. In either case a mixed infection will occur, and a suppurating track is likely to remain for some weeks.

In the chronic types, prostatic massage *per rectum*, with the occasional passage of a large metal sound or Kollmann's dilator under local anaesthesia should be carried out.

Instillation into the posterior urethra of 5 per cent. collargol is often beneficial. It can be carried out once or twice a week, 2 drachms being sufficient. It is introduced by means of the Canny Ryall syringe, and should be retained for 10 min. at least.

The subacute type of prostatitis, associated with *B. coli* infection of the urine, is most satisfactorily treated by prostatic massage carried out daily to begin with, and the administration of a urinary antiseptic—pyridium or neotropine being, in this type, the most efficacious. Cherry-stalk tea or barley water should be taken, and alcoholic and venereal excess forbidden. Strychnine in the form of strychnine sulphate or nitrate gr. 1/20 given as a pill three times a day is very beneficial. Diathermy *per rectum* occasionally helps.

In these cases treatment is very satisfactory, but the condition is apt to recur—a fact of which the patient should be made aware.

CALCULUS

Calculi in the prostate are not uncommon, and often un-associated with symptoms. They are most commonly dis-covered after a routine radiological examination. They consist of phosphate, oxalate or carbonate of calcium, and are opaque to the X-rays. They are usually small in size but are often present in large numbers, although a single large calculus may occur.

The symptoms are those of a basal cystitis. In association with prostatic enlargement they may cause difficulty in micturition and retention of urine. Haematuria sometimes occurs, and the calculus may be palpable *per rectum* or on the passage of a sound. Prostatic calculi practically always throw a shadow on the X-ray plate.

Treatment. When calculi are giving rise to symptoms they should be removed. This may be carried out by the suprapubic or perineal route—more rarely by means of the Bumpus punch or the operating cysto-urethroscope introduced into the urethra.

TUBERCULOSIS OF THE PROSTATE

See chapter IX on Genito-urinary Tuberculosis.

CHRONIC ENLARGEMENT OF THE PROSTATE

(Syn. senile hypertrophy, adenoma of the prostate, fibro-adenoma of the prostate, fibromyoma of the prostate, simple enlargement)

This clinical condition, as may be gathered from its large number of synonyms, covers a variety of pathological forms. It occurs most frequently between the ages of 50 and 70, and is characterized by a benign enlargement of the prostate, which makes its presence felt by interference with the mechanism of micturition.

From the fortieth year of life onwards the prostate increases slightly in size, but this enlargement is not pathological, is unaccompanied by symptoms, and is merely the normal expression of an ageing gland. It should, however, be borne in mind lest the inexperienced fall into the error of attributing the physiological enlargement of this organ to pathological changes.

Aetiology. The causes of pathological enlargement of the prostate are unknown, to a large extent unsuspected, and the theories of these causes at the moment entirely unproved. Sexual excesses, alcoholism and infections—particularly with the gonococcus—have all received their share of condemnation. There is some evidence, however, that the "fibrous" prostate carries a more frequent antecedent history of gonorrhoea than the glandular type of enlargement.

Riches and Muir, investigating cases of prostatic enlargement at the Middlesex Hospital, found that in those cases of enlargement which gave a history of gonorrhoea, fibrosis occurred in 47 per cent., while in those cases of enlargement which did not give this venereal history, fibrosis occurred in only 26 per cent. of cases.

That it is an involutionary process occurring in an organ no longer functioning, is merely a method of expressing the well-known fact that it occurs after the prime of life, without attempting to state a cause.

Pathology. Benign enlargements of the prostate fall clinically into three groups:

       (1) The large, soft prostate (adenoma).

       (2) The "fibrous" prostate.

       (3) The calculous prostate.

Large, Soft Prostate

In the first type the lateral and middle lobes bear the brunt of enlargement, the anterior and posterior lobes being comparatively rarely affected. This is the type often referred to as the large, soft prostate, and, though variable in size, is not uncommonly as big as a tangerine or even a cricket ball.

Enlargement of the lateral lobes may be felt *per rectum*, but an intravesical enlargement of the "middle" lobe ("prostatic bar") may occur independent of any marked enlargement on the part of the lateral lobes. Again, the periurethral part of the prostate may project into the bladder to form a well-marked "collar". Both the "median bar" and the "prostatic collar" are impalpable *per rectum*, and can only be demonstrated prior to operation by cystoscopic examination. The pathological process most commonly responsible for this enlargement consists of a collection of nodules of glandular tissue which by their growth compress the surrounding tissue and give rise to the familiar "adenoma". These nodules are made up of cystic acini lying in a fibromuscular stroma. Close to the urethra, muscle fibre may be in evidence and occasionally in excess, so that in the past these tumours have been thought to resemble the fibromyomata of the uterus.

Pari passu with the increase of acini in the "middle" and lateral lobes, the posterior lobe is compressed and often stretched over the posterior part of the enlarged prostate as a thin layer of atrophic cells. There is evidence to support the view that this atrophy of the posterior lobe is not the result of compression by the enlarging periurethral part of the prostate, but rather a possible cause of it. Atrophy in the posterior lobe generally antedates the enlargements of the "middle" and lateral lobes of the prostate. This might possibly lead to a loss of balance and restraint on the part of the periurethral areas, with a consequent unimpeded over-growth, when the normal posterior lobe undergoes regression.

Fibrous Prostate

In this condition the prostate is generally small, hard, without intravesical prominences, and consists of a tissue in which the glandular elements are few and an interstitial fibrosis forms the bulk of the organ. Fibrous nodules occur in the position of previous acini, and in the periurethral muscular sheath. Perivascular lymphocytosis is usually present.

Calculous Prostate

Small calculi may be present in any part of the gland, but the term "calculous prostate" generally refers to a fibrotic condition of the gland, associated with well-marked calculi which may be numerous, and are not limited to any one lobe. A history of some urethral infection is common.

From this brief consideration of the pathology of prostatic enlargement it is obvious that the prostate owes its clinical importance solely to its position surrounding the outlet of the bladder. By its growth and interference with the process of micturition morbid changes take place in the associated urinary organs and elsewhere. These may be considered under the headings:
(1) Urethra.
(2) The bladder.
(3) Upper urinary tract.
(4) Sexual organs.
(5) Cardio-vascular system.
(6) Mentality.

(1) Urethra

The prostate enlarges upwards as the rigid triangular liga-ments preclude its extension towards the perineum. The urethra is therefore lengthened—often by one or more inches

—and its lumen altered in calibre by distortions of the lateral lobes. If there is much enlargement of the "middle" lobe, the posterior wall of the urethra above the common ejaculatory ducts will be so lengthened that the normal prostatic curve becomes converted to a rectangle, the point of which corresponds with—and is to a certain extent anchored by—the entry of the common ejaculatory ducts. The substitution

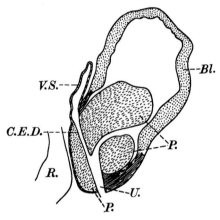

Fig. 29. Diagrammatic section of bladder and enlarged prostate to show rectangularity of urethra. *Bl.*, Bladder. *C.E.D.*, Common ejaculatory duct. *P.,P.,P.*, Prostate. *R.*, Rectum. *U.*, Prostatic urethra. *V.S.*, Vesicula seminalis.

of this rectangle for the normal curve results in an increased difficulty in both micturition and the passage of a catheter (Fig. 29).

(2) *The Bladder*

Changes in this organ take the form, in the early stages, of a compensatory hypertrophy of the bladder wall. Concurrently with this, trabeculation becomes marked, and the trigonal muscle prominent as a hypertrophied ridge along the base of the bladder. Small pouches and diverticula become manifest in which stone formation is not uncommon. So long as the bladder by its muscular hypertrophy is able to overcome the increasing difficulty in micturition, a thick-walled "compensated" organ (comparable with the heart in similar conditions) results.

When retention takes place or failure of compensation is initiated, the bladder dilates, the muscular wall becomes thinner, and a "failing" bladder results. Residual urine increases in amount, or retention and overflow may take place. Micturition lacks force, or the stream may be reduced to a trickle. The mucous membrane becomes hyperaemic, and sooner or later infection with the production of a cystitis—basal or general—results.

(3) *Upper Urinary Tract*

In some cases enlargement of the prostate is accompanied by dilatation of the ureter and renal pelvis—often bilateral. This was formerly believed to be due to direct "back pressure" on the upper urinary tract by the obstruction to the urinary outflow occasioned by the diseased prostate.

On examination of the ureters in these cases, although they may be greatly enlarged and hydronephrosis well marked at their upper extremity, their lower orifice is in most cases normal, and only rarely is it widely open. Furthermore, the very oblique course of the ureter through the bladder wall would seem to preclude the possibility of urinary backflow from this organ to the upper urinary tract taking place.

It is more probable that in those cases in which marked hypertrophy of the vesical musculature occurs obstruction to the **lower end of the ureter** results from this increased muscular development and possible spasm round the ureteric orifice, with a consequent hindrance to the effective emptying of the renal pelvis and ureter, rather than a dilatation in continuity of the whole urinary tract above the urethra.

Whatever the precise cause of ureteric and renal dilatation may be, the result is the development, in some cases, of a bilateral hydronephrosis, in others an interstitial nephritis, and in both an impairment or failure of renal function which may progress to uraemia and death.

(4) *Sexual Organs*

Compression or distortion of the common ejaculatory ducts takes place and aspermia results. Frequent erections are common, and an insatiable sexual appetite may be developed. Orchitis occasionally occurs, although it is rare until instrumentation or operation has taken place.

(5) *Cardio-vascular System*

The veins around the prostate in continuity with those of the bladder, and the dorsal vein of the penis, enlarge, and may sometimes rupture with the formation of a profuse haematuria or excessive bruising of penis and perineum. Arteriosclerosis is common in the later stages.

(6) *Mentality*

Changes in the mentality of the individual afflicted with a large prostate may take the form of acts of gross impropriety, distressing alike both to the patient and his relatives. A pre vious impotence may give place to excessive venery.

Symptoms. *Rarely*, prostatic enlargement first makes itself evident by an attack of acute urinary retention, or a condition of retention and overflow is discovered by the doctor. Still more rarely, a bout of haematuria may be the first intimation of prostatic hypertrophy. Occasionally priapism, or a marked change in the patient's sexual appetite, suggests to him, or his doctor, a possible prostatic cause.

Commonly, the first symptom is increased frequency of micturition which, though it may pass unnoticed during the day, generally forces its attention on the patient when getting him out of bed two or more times during the night. With this increase in frequency, difficulty—at first slight but later becoming marked—in commencing the act is noticed. Straining often makes matters worse, as in those cases in which enlargement of the "middle" lobe has taken place with the production of a rectangular urethra, it is apt to constrict still further the already kinked urethra by forcing its posterior wall downwards. Frequently the patient mentions this fact, and volunteers the statement that only by a placid avoidance of all hurry is he able to initiate the act at all. With the progress of the enlargement a stream diminished both in volume and projectile force results, and the patient often complains of his inability to keep the lower parts of his trousers dry when making water owing to this failure of projection.

Pain is not a marked symptom until cystitis supervenes or retention occurs, but a feeling of discomfort in perineum and rectum is sometimes mentioned.

Haematuria may occur, but is not a common symptom apart from instrumentation. Occasionally during the administration of a local anaesthetic (detailed in chapter II), and prior to the introduction of any instrument *per urethram*, the effect of massaging the fluid to the posterior urethra may result in the production of a few drops of blood at the external meatus—particularly when the prostate is soft and highly engorged. In a few cases haematuria may be a prominent symptom, and clots may fill the bladder, necessitating prolonged irrigation before cystoscopy can be undertaken. The occurrence of such marked haemorrhage, however, should not fail to raise the suspicion of some other condition, e.g. vesical papilloma or carcinoma being present in addition to the simple prostatic enlargement.

With the progress of the disease residual urine increases,

and "back pressure" symptoms make their appearance on the upper urinary tract. Signs of renal involvement such as thirst, headache, hiccup or vomiting, together with a high blood urea and low urea concentration, indicate an advanced condition complicated by damage to the secretory mechanism of the body.

Sooner or later infection occurs with the production of a foul cystitis, and very often development of vesical calculi. Attacks of acute retention may occur and are commonly induced by cold, holding the urine too long, or following alcohol or other excesses.

In the unsuspected and untreated cases chronic retention and overflow is often found. This may be quite painless in some cases—the patient merely complaining that he is always making water—while in others a persistent dribbling, associated with oedema of penis and scrotum together with pain and permanently wet clothing, is found. In both a distended bladder can be made out on palpation above the pubis.

In late cases signs of impairment of the general health become marked: loss of sleep and appetite, together with increased thirst, vomiting and headache, are present. The cardio-vascular and pulmonary systems become affected, with danger to the patient's life.

Investigation. The investigation of these cases has in view two main objects:

    (1) The diagnosis.

    (2) The type of treatment necessary.

The diagnosis is simple. A patient of over 50 years of age who presents signs of commencing urinary obstruction possesses almost certainly an enlarged prostate or urethral stricture. Rectal examination will reveal enlargement of the lateral and posterior lobes, but the "middle lobe" is not palpable from this aspect. The enlargement is smooth, regular and moderately soft in consistency in the adenomatous types.

The cleft between the two lateral lobes can sometimes be felt, one lobe often being larger than the other. Occasionally harder nodules may be present, representing isolated fibro-adenomata or calculi.

A smaller and harder prostate will be present where fibrosis is marked, while the typical prostate of malignant disease gives to the feeling of the examining finger a sensation of inelasticity and stony hardness.

The rectal mucous membrane should move freely across the simple enlarged prostate, but may be fixed and infiltrated in advanced cases of malignant disease.

Unless contraindicated by symptoms of extreme urgency from renal or cardiac failure, or the presence of some impassable urethral obstruction, cystoscopy should always be carried out. Hindrance to the passage of this instrument in the region of the prostate may be noticed, and its proximal end may need extreme depression between the patient's thighs before it can be made to enter the bladder. Through it can be seen hypertrophy of the "middle lobe", or the elevated "collar" of periurethral and intravesical prostatic enlargement. It is not gripped tightly by the prostate either on introduction or withdrawal as in a stricture.

Isolated nodules in the upper surface of the prostate can be inspected; the amount of residual urine can be estimated at the same time, and the presence of calculi or growth determined.

Attention directed to the walls of the bladder will bring to light the degree of trabeculation, and whether or not pouches or diverticula are present.

An inspection of the base may show a well-marked ridge due to hypertrophy of the trigonal muscle and the condition of the ureteric orifices can be noted.

In cases of fibrous prostate there may be little or no intra-vesical enlargement, and the passage of a urethroscope may be necessary to determine the amount of constriction at the internal urinary meatus.

Radiology is valuable, as a calculous prostate can be demonstrated thereby, or it may be needed to demonstrate the size of a diverticulum after its previous filling with opaque fluid.

Before any treatment of the enlarged prostate is undertaken a bacteriological examination of the urine is advisable, and an enquiry as to the degree of renal competence is essential. (Tests of Renal Functions, chapter i.)

Treatment. Before discussing the treatment of the enlarged prostate it may not be out of place briefly to consider the methods in vogue during the past 30 years.

Formerly, the unhappy possessors of enlarged prostates which gave rise to urinary retention carried on existence by means of catheter life, or submitted to an operation which carried a very high mortality. This latter, although reduced by careful selection of cases and by suitable preliminary treatment, is still too high, and varies greatly according to whether the statistics be those of general surgeons or urologists, and again between private and hospital types of case.

The earlier operations for removal of the prostate were carried out via the perineum—a method never very popular in England, and even in the United States now finding few adherents.

Later the operation popularized by Freyer, which consists of an intravesical removal of the adenomatous prostate, was practised almost universally. Although giving admirable results in the hands of the expert, this operation as practised by the less skilled carried in its wake a terribly high mortality —probably due in many cases to the unsatisfactory type of case on which the operation was performed. Still later, efficient preliminary treatment and the performance of the operation in two stages effected a reduction in the mortality.

Nevertheless the great bugbears of shock, haemorrhage and sepsis remained to carry off many cases that would otherwise have been free to continue in normal life. In certain cases too, post-operative obstruction would occur, due to excessive fibrosis and contracture round the bladder outlet.

With a view to overcoming the serious and not uncommonly fatal handicap of excessive haemorrhage, various methods were introduced, e.g. plugging the prostatic cavity with gauze, or the introduction of a hydrostatic bag into the prostatic cavity continuous with a urethral catheter.

Modifications in the operative procedure next made their appearance, following the methods of Thompson Walker or some variation of them. In order to prevent post-operative obstruction, and the better to control haemorrhage, visualization of the prostatic pouch after digital removal of the gland was practised. By suitable retractors the inside of the bladder could be well shown and the opening from bladder to prostatic pouch demonstrated. In order to prevent ledge formation and to throw bladder and pouch into one cavity, some operators excised a wedge from the posterior lip of the cavity: others, perhaps wiser in their generation, omitted this step. At any rate all bleeding points that could be controlled with forceps or ligature were so dealt with, and by means of a continuous suture of the mucous membrane round the prostatic pouch, a marked lessening of haemorrhage was assured. The extra time necessary for the operation was considerable, and in many cases shock was marked.

In 1930 Sir John Thompson Walker, in his Lettsomian Lectures, gave the operative mortality of prostatectomy at 19·5 per cent., which fact he derived from the study of the statistics of some twelve general hospitals. There is ample evidence for believing that this figure is by no means too high an estimation.

About this time attempts to lower this mortality were

taking the form of perurethral methods, by which means areas of the prostate were subjected to the diathermic current with a resultant coagulation and necrosis of their tissues (fulguration). Although this method was applicable to only a few types of prostate, and carried with it a high septic morbidity, promising results were chronicled—notably from France.

At the present time, the evolution of prostatic surgery is proceeding along two divergent lines: on the one hand are attempts towards a more extensive type of prostatectomy, having as their aim an immediate reconstruction of the urethra and a closure of the bladder, culminating in the operation practised by Harris, of Sydney; on the other hand are found efforts to reduce all operative procedure to the minimum, with the removal through the urethra of the obstructing parts of the prostate by endothermic resection—carried out by means of a resectoscope of the McCarthy type.

From this brief survey it is obvious that there is not entire agreement on the part of urologists and general surgeons as to the ideal treatment of prostatic enlargement, and though all are agreed that the aim of treatment is to remove once and for all the barrier to free and effective urination, opinions differ as to the best method of effecting this aim.

As has been seen, enlargement of the prostate may be complicated by a variety of conditions, and such concomitants as severe cystitis, the presence of vesical calculi, or an infected pouch, will obviously need removal as a first step towards treatment of the prostate. Cases of marked renal impairment with high blood urea (over 50 mg. per 100 c.c.), or low urea concentration (less than 2 per cent. in the second hour), are distinctly bad risks for prostatectomy until the renal mechanism has regained to some extent its normal function following prolonged catheter drainage or suprapubic cystostomy.

Furthermore, cases of acute retention should not be submitted to prostatectomy until the patient has not only recovered from that attack of acute retention (if necessary relieved and afterwards prevented by the use of the catheter), but has also shown himself to be the possessor of adequately functioning kidneys.

Retention with overflow almost invariably demands a preliminary cystostomy if the prostate is to be removed with a reasonable degree of safety. In many—if not most—cases in which a preliminary drainage of the bladder is desired in order to improve renal function or overcome severe cystitis, catheter drainage will be found to be difficult or inadvisable. Few individuals tolerate well the frequent passage of a catheter over long periods, and permanent drainage by an indwelling catheter too often gives rise to a severe urethritis, with the consequent absorption of toxins.

In these cases suprapubic cystotomy, performed at the highest point of the distended bladder, should be carried out. Drainage must be maintained until the urine is practically clear, and the renal function considered adequate to withstand further operative strain. A daily bladder wash with 1/6000 oxycyanide of mercury is helpful in keeping the bladder clean, but when marked cystitis is present silver nitrate solution 1/2000, increasing in strength, is generally more effective.

For those cases of enlarged prostate, uncomplicated by severe cystitis, calculi or marked renal impairment, English opinion at the present day is in general agreement that the large, soft (adenomatous) prostate is best treated by suprapubic removal. Ideally, this should be performed by the method of Harris, in which the prostatic cavity is obliterated round a catheter and the bladder closed (described in next chapter). In the hands of its inventor this operation has a mortality of less than 2·7 per cent.—a figure which is unlikely to be attained by any but the most skilled, and only after due attention to case selection, and efficient preliminary treatment. In very old men, and bad surgical risks, however, the extra time and shock of this operation may incline one to adopt the much more rapid method of Freyer.

Again where a preliminary cystostomy has been performed, owing to the induration of the tissues about the wound considerable difficulty may be experienced in providing sufficient space for effective visualization of the prostatic cavity, and the method of Harris may be impracticable.

There will be few dissenters from the view that fibrous prostates, and those with a prominent "middle lobe" without much enlargement of the lateral lobes, are most satisfactorily treated by the perurethral method of resection with the McCarthy or Canny Ryall resectoscope.

Between the fairly clear-cut groups of the large, soft prostates on the one hand, and the fibrous and "median bar" types on the other, are the vast majority which call for treatment; and it is this large collection of different types, occurring in individuals of widely different ages, and varying renal function, that are responsible for the divergent views of urologists to-day.

The chief problem is presented by the moderately enlarged adenomatous prostate, in the individual of poor general condition and with considerable impairment of renal function. On the one hand, by preliminary drainage (by catheter, or more usually cystostomy), this type of case may be rendered reasonably safe for the performance of a prostatectomy at a later date, while on the other hand perurethral resection of the prostate may be carried out on one or more occasions without the necessity of preliminary bladder drainage, and with a very much enhanced chance of survival.

It should be mentioned in passing that approximately 80 per cent. of operations on the prostate at the Mayo Clinic take the form of this latter method of treatment, the mortality of which is practically negligible, and certainly much less than 1 per cent.

To sum up, prostatectomy is the method of choice in large, and very large, soft prostates, although a preliminary cystostomy may be necessary in certain cases before the prostate can be removed.

Perurethral resection is indicated in cases of fibrous prostate, prostates with a prominent "middle lobe" unassociated with marked lateral lobe enlargement, and also in those cases of poor general condition in which the performance of a prostatectomy would be a serious risk.

Furthermore, those cases with marked general enlargement which were formerly adjudged suitable only for a permanent suprapubic cystostomy—by reason of poor general condition —may nowadays be given the benefit of endoscopic resection without the attendant discomfort of a permanent suprapubic fistula even if, in some few cases, it might need repeating on one or more occasions.

Preliminary Surgical Treatment. As has already been mentioned, in cases where calculi, marked cystitis, or infected pouches are present, these will need rectifying before operation on the prostate takes place. Preliminary treatment in these cases will take the form of suprapubic cystostomy, the removal of the calculi, and removal or drainage of an infected pouch. In a few cases a pouch may be rendered clean by cystoscopic lavage, and the filling of its cavity with liquid paraffin. More generally it will need excision, or enlargement of its opening into the bladder by incision.

Cases in which the blood urea is over 50 mg. per 100 c.c., or urea concentration below 2 per cent. in the second hour, or in which the excretion of intravenous indigo-carmine is poor, will need preliminary bladder drainage by an indwelling catheter, or cystostomy. When a catheter is used every effort towards surgical cleanliness must be made, and the catheter changed every other day, the urethra being washed out at the change of catheter.

Bladder washes, as in cystostomy, may be necessary, and the catheter drainage should be continued until renal function is satisfactory or the urethra becomes too inflamed to tolerate the presence of this foreign body. In the event of the latter occurrence, if renal efficiency is still considered inadequate, cystostomy must be performed. When this becomes necessary the opening should be made at the highest point in the bladder, and an interval of at least one month should elapse before prostatectomy is carried out in order to allow of the subsidence of induration round the wound.

Endoscopic resection, on the other hand, may be undertaken as soon as the renal efficiency is adjudged satisfactory.

Cases of acute retention, or of retention and overflow resulting in a distended bladder, will need gradual "decompression" lest anuria or haemorrhage result from a too rapid emptying of the vesical contents. This may be effected in a variety of ways but the outlet of urine should be so regulated that not more than 4 oz. per hour are withdrawn.

Vas ligation and vasectomy are practised as a routine by some surgeons preparatory to prostatectomy, as postoperative epididymitis is extremely common. Winsbury White has placed this as high as 82 per cent. Other surgeons, including the writer, while not denying the prevalence of this complication, feel that it is easier to observe and deal with inflammation in a comparatively superficial organ like the testis, rather than face the probability of infection and suppuration in such a deep-seated structure as the vesicula seminalis, which may result from the damming back of infected matter by ligature of the vas.

Before any operation on the prostate, suitable pre-operative measures as to disinfection of the urine and attention to sterilization of skin and penis must of course be carried out.

POST-OPERATIVE COMPLICATIONS AND SEQUELAE

The post-operative complications of prostatectomy and prostate resection are the chief bugbears of these operations. They take the form of shock, haemorrhage (primary and secondary), extravasation of urine, and sepsis about the wound and in more distant organs, e.g. epididymis or kidney. More remotely, obstruction to the normal passage of urine, incontinence of urine, and the persistence of a suprapubic fistula have to be reckoned with, while the formation of calculi in the bladder or prostatic pouch have not been uncommon in the past.

Primary Haemorrhage

Primary haemorrhage should not occur after Harris's operation, owing to the careful attention to haemostasis. It is rare for it to be of any magnitude after perurethral operations, and when it does occur, urethral irrigation, the tying in of a catheter, or the visualization of the bleeding point by urethroscopy and its searing by a touch with the diathermy electrode will control it. Primary haemorrhage, on the other hand, is not uncommon after prostatectomy has been performed by Freyer's method, and less commonly after Thompson Walker's operation. Douching with hot saline (temp. 130° F.) will usually control it, while some surgeons prefer to plug the prostatic pouch with gauze which can be gradually removed from 48 to 56 hours after the operation. Others prefer to make use of the hydrostatic bag of Fullerton or Pilcher type. These are most easily inserted by passing a sound through the urethra to the bladder to which the catheter-like tube of the bag is attached and withdrawn through the urethra to the outside. The bag is distended with fluid, and the tube attached to a weight of 2 lb. over the end of the bed. It can be maintained in position for 48 hours. It is apt to give rise to a good deal of discomfort, and the writer is of opinion that after 8–10 hours it should be emptied of its contents and relieved of its extension weight (unless haemorrhage is still continuing), but not removed from the bladder until 48 hours have elapsed since the operation. It can then be refilled and the weight attached again at the first sign of recommencement of haemorrhage.

Secondary Haemorrhage

Secondary haemorrhage is due to sepsis, and commonly occurs 7–10 days after operation. It is of grave import, may be very profuse and very depressing to the patient. Morphia, haemostatic serum, hot douching and intramuscular calcium should all be tried, whilst blood transfusion may become necessary. If it is not rapidly controlled by these methods the bladder must be reopened and attempts made to deal with the bleeding point by ligature or compression, after which the suprapubic opening in the bladder should be left widely open and not stitched up tightly round a tube.

Extravasation of Urine

This is a very serious condition, but fortunately is not common nowadays. It is liable to occur into the cave of Retzius and round the neck of the bladder in cases where, for any reason, the bladder is not stitched tightly round the suprapubic tube, and where leakage has occurred into the perivesical tissues. It rapidly gives rise to a highly septic, and generally foul smelling, condition in which large sloughs may be prominent, and the general condition of the patient may quickly deteriorate. Very rarely it may occur from the sloughing of the prostate after the too thorough application of the endothermic electrode, in which case an artificial opening into the rectum may occur. Owing to the highly irritating and septic nature of the extravasated urine, a thorough and complete opening up of the infected areas must be carried out as early as possible.

Sepsis

Sepsis takes the form of wound infection, cystitis, or infections of various organs at a distance, e.g. the vesiculae seminales, epididymis and the kidney. These should be treated on the principles laid down under their separate headings.

Obstruction and Incontinence of Urine

Obstruction to the normal outflow of urine was formerly not uncommon after the operation of prostatectomy. It was usually due to a fibrosis taking place at the bladder outlet, or to damage to the membraneous urethra after a too radical removal of the prostate. It is much less common nowadays owing to the inception of Harris's operation, or to the earlier passage of sounds, and efficient dilatation after the other types of prostatectomy.

It is most satisfactorily treated by the administration of a local anaesthetic, and the dilatation of the bladder outlet by a curved Kollmann's dilator. Occasionally the constriction rapidly reforms, and it may be necessary to enlarge the internal urinary meatus by applications of the diathermy electrode introduced through the urethroscope, this procedure generally calling for spinal, caudal or general anaesthesia.

Following the use of the resectoscope, stricture of the urethra is not uncommon—generally at the external meatus or in the prostate. It is due to the trauma inflicted on the urethra by the large resectoscope. It should be treated by the passage of sounds or meatal dilators, and the likelihood of its occurrence after this type of operation must ever be in mind.

Post-operative incontinence is generally present for a short while after prostatectomy. It usually clears up in a few days or weeks, but occasionally persists. It is generally associated with a too extensive removal of the prostate, which may have included the verumontanum and the anterior commissure.

Urethroscopy shows an incompetent sphincter vesicae, and unless the sphincter urethrae membranaceae can be encouraged to act more vigorously, incontinence is likely to remain. Hot douching of the urethra, massage to the bladder neck *per rectum*, tonics and occasional rectal diathermy may alleviate or cure the condition. Where no treatment is of avail, a permanent urinal worn on the thigh and fixed to the penis may become necessary.

Persistence, or Undue Delay in Healing of a Suprapubic Fistula

This condition is fortunately not common nowadays. It may be due to gross urinary sepsis, often associated with the presence of calculi, or an infected pouch—which conditions will need treatment or removal before the fistulous track can be expected to heal.

The second, and perhaps commonest cause of delayed healing of the suprapubic wound is obstruction at the bladder neck, the removal of which (by dilatation or diathermy) generally suffices to clear up the condition.

Where gross sepsis and obstruction at the bladder neck are absent the insertion of a catheter *per urethram* and retained *in situ* may promote healing; while yet other cases—particularly if there is reason to suppose there is a mucous or skin lining to the fistula—will call for opening up of the suprapubic wound and excision of the fistulous track.

Post-operative Calculi

Post-operative calculi are liable to occur if there has been much sepsis, and are not very uncommon following fulguration of the prostate, and after partial resection of that organ with the resectoscope. Particularly are they liable to occur when portions of the prostate are inadvertently left behind instead of being removed on the endothermic wire. Their presence calls for crushing or removal.

AFTER-CARE OF THE PROSTATIC CASE

All patients after any operation on the prostate should be subjected to review at periodic intervals during the first year after their discharge from hospital.

Such conditions as persistent cystitis, bladder-neck obstructions, stone formation or renal insufficiency can then be observed and treated at the earliest possible moment: while after the use of the resectoscope a urethral or external meatal stricture not uncommonly develops (probably owing to the large size of the instrument) which can be easily rectified by the use of a meatal dilator.

It cannot be too strongly emphasized that after severe operations on the prostate, however normal may appear the urinary apparatus, the mental capacity of the individual may take many months to regain its normal vigour, and excessive brain work should be strongly discouraged for 6 months, at least, after the operation.

NEW GROWTHS OF THE PROSTATE

These may take the form of sarcoma or carcinoma. Sarcoma is extremely rare, many cases previously so described being in fact carcinomata of an atypical type.

CARCINOMA

Pathologically carcinoma of the prostate is characterized by the excessive polymorphism of its cells. It may be of a schirrus or medullary type, according to the amount of fibrous tissue present.

Clinically three types of carcinomata occur, each with signs and symptoms peculiar to its own group:

Group 1. "Latent type." This type occurs in prostates having the characteristics of simple enlargement, which may be removed under the impression that they are benign, until a microscopic investigation brings to light a deep seated area with malignant characteristics. Dissemination is not marked, and if it occurs is limited to the local lymph drainage. A relatively good prognosis after operation in these cases may be given.

Group 2. "Invasive type." In this type growth is rapid, and extends away from the prostate in all directions—fungating into bladder and rectum, and encroaching along the pelvic floor to involve the pelvic glands to the hollow of the sacrum. These cases include the diffuse prostato-pelvic carcinomas of Guyon. In addition to urinary signs pain is a marked feature, and is generally felt in and about the pelvis and along the sciatic nerves. It has been attributed to invasion by the growth of the sacral plexus, cauda equina, and pelvic bones.

Group 3. "Metastatic." Cases of this type possess few urinary symptoms but give rise to diffuse metastases in bone, often far distant from the prostate. The vertebrae and the femur below the middle are perhaps most commonly attacked, but humerus, clavicle and skull, or rib, are not uncommonly the seat of secondary deposits. Spontaneous fracture may occur. In this group the spread of carcinoma is difficult to understand, and may be due to a blood dissemination, or, as Roberts suggests, to an invasion of the lymph spaces about the spinal column—particularly along the laminae and ligamenta flava. It has been thought that carcinoma cells carried either by permeation or embolism to the region of the anterior sacral foramena might thereafter ascend the lymph and tissue spaces around the spinal cord to the upper parts of the body. It must, however, be admitted that there is somewhat meagre evidence for this hypothesis.

Signs and Symptoms. In Group 1 the signs and symptoms are those of simple enlargement of the prostate.

In Group 2, in addition to the signs of simple enlargement (i.e. frequency, and difficulty of micturition), pain is often marked—particularly in the pelvis and down the thighs, due to the involvement of the sacral plexus by the spreading carcinoma—and occasionally true incontinence may occur from involvement of the bladder sphincters. Haematuria is not a marked feature unless ulceration occurs, in which case it will be associated with pyuria. In more advanced cases invasion of the rectum, progressing to fistula formation, may occur. Retention is common and enlargement of the inguinal glands has been noticed.

Digital examination, *per rectum*, reveals an enlarged, stony-hard and nodular gland, often with irregular prolongations of induration at the sides of the rectum. The mucous membrane may be tightly attached to the tumour, and bimanually considerable fixity of the bladder may be made out.

Cystoscopy is not a great help to diagnosis in these cases except to demonstrate the presence of ulceration, but an X-ray may be invaluable, particularly if the pelvic bones are the seat of secondary deposits.

In Group 3, the first intimation may be a spontaneous fracture of the thigh or humerus. More commonly the patient complains of vague pain or discomfort, or a bony swelling may be noted.

An X-ray will show carcinomatous involvement of the bones, but there may be few signs to connect the prostate with these secondary manifestations. As a rule the prostate is slightly enlarged and harder than usual, but obstructive signs are few or absent.

Treatment. Except in cases of Group 1, curative treatment is perhaps less hopeful than anywhere else in the body. Suprapubic or perineal removal is rapidly followed by a recurrence. Deep X-ray therapy, although it often relieves the pain, has little curative effect on the carcinoma. Nor has radium, either in the shape of radon seeds or in the form of radium element, fulfilled its early hopes.

Two types of palliative treatment, on the other hand, have met with considerable success. Where pain is a marked feature and is unrelieved by X-ray therapy, section of the presacral nerve is often followed by marked alleviation. If urinary retention is the chief concern, a permanent suprapubic cystotomy may be necessary. Fortunately, however, this contingency is becoming rarer, and an effective passage through the prostate can usually be assured by the aid of the resectoscope. Indeed, one of the great advantages of this most useful instrument is its ability to save the doomed patient from the additional distress of a suprapubic fistula.

NEUROSES

Prostatic neuroses take the form of hypersensibility, urinary incontinence, spasmodic retention, and certain varieties of impotence, and are most commonly found in young adults.

In the first type pain or discomfort may be noticed in the perineum, and rectal examination reveals an extremely tender prostate—raising perhaps a suspicion of an infective prostatitis. The urine, however, is free from organisms, no discharge is present and the temperature is normal.

Premature ejaculation of semen, amounting to impotence, is commonly associated, and urethroscopic examination shows an enlarged and sensitive verumontanum.

In the spasmodic types difficulty is experienced in commencing micturition, which can often only be effected in entire seclusion and after a considerable delay. There is, however, no obstruction to the passage of a catheter, nor is the prostate enlarged.

In cases in which urinary incontinence is the predominant feature, atony of the prostate has been blamed, and urethroscopic examination reveals a poorly contracting sphincter vesicae. This incontinence is generally partial, resulting in urinary leakage at the beginning and end of micturition, but the main bulk of urine is held unless some sudden psychic stimulation occurs, necessitating urgent emptying of the bladder. Impotence may occur.

Treatment. In the hyperaesthetic type, hot fomentations or hip baths, together with the administration of bromides, may be of use. Prostatic massage, although resented, is sometimes helpful. Topical applications of silver nitrate to the posterior urethra, by means of the urethroscope, should be tried in those cases of functional impotence associated with a prominent and tender verumontanum.

Patients, in whom difficulty of micturition is marked, should be treated by the frequent passage of a large sound or Kollmann's dilator, while the atonic types derive the greatest benefit from prostatic massage, strychnine and occasional topical applications of collargol or silver nitrate to the posterior urethra.

Chapter XII

OPERATIONS ON THE PROSTATE

Operations on the prostate may be carried out through a suprapubic cystotomy, e.g. Freyer's, Thompson Walker's, and Harris's methods, or *per urethram* by means of the urethroscope as in fulguration and resection of the prostate.

SUPRAPUBIC PROSTATECTOMY
METHOD OF FREYER

This method, which held sway for many years, consists in the rapid enucleation of the prostate by the finger and the insertion of a rubber tube into the suprapubic opening in the bladder. It can be carried out very rapidly in cases of adenomatous enlargement, but is apt to be followed by severe haemorrhage, and may be associated with unnecessary removal of a large part of the urethra. It is perhaps most useful in cases presenting a large, soft prostate, in association with old age, which would ill withstand the strain of a more prolonged operation. In cases in which a preliminary cystotomy has already been carried out it may be the only method applicable for prostatectomy at a later date.

Suprapubic cystotomy having been performed, the right index finger defines the prostate and breaks through the mucous membrane at the internal urinary meatus. By passing round the anterior, lateral and posterior lobes, the prostate is separated from its pouch. If any difficulty is experienced in this the index finger of the opposite hand, or that of an assistant, may be placed in the rectum in order to push the prostate upwards, which hand for convenience sake should be fitted with two gloves—the outer glove being removed on withdrawal of the finger from the rectum.

The adenoma having been delivered, the bladder and prostatic pouch are irrigated with hot antiseptic introduced through the suprapubic wound (or by means of a catheter), with a view both to controlling haemorrhage and promoting contraction of the prostatic pouch. Should haemorrhage persist, the introduction of plugging or the hydrostatic bag into the prostatic pouch will be called for.

A large suprapubic drainage tube, through which irrigation can be carried out, is left *in situ* for 10 days—the bladder wall having been closely stitched round it.

If the tube is left some 6 in. long, a suitable connection can be made so that urine can be drained into a reservoir attached to the side of the bed—the patient's comfort being thereby greatly enhanced.

After 10 days the suprapubic tube can be removed and a Hamilton Irving box substituted. If the patient has not passed water naturally by the twelfth day, a catheter passed *per urethram* will usually assist the closure of the suprapubic wound. At any sign of urethral obstruction the passage of a large metal sound or Kollmann's dilator should be instigated.

METHOD OF THOMPSON WALKER

In this method the preliminary steps are identical with those of the previous method, except that the incision of abdominal wall and bladder is longer—generally reaching from umbilicus to pubis.

After the enucleation of the prostate a large retractor is inserted in order to visualize the prostatic pouch. In the earlier operations by this method a V-shaped portion of tissue lying between the two ureters was excised from the prostatic rim in order to prevent ledge formation between the empty prostatic cavity and the bladder. Many operators nowadays omit this step on the ground that it still further opens up tissues liable to infection, and moreover is apt to damage or remove the trigonal muscle with the resultant impairment of post-operative micturition.

A continuous suture is then inserted between the mucous membrane and the prostatic pouch, which generally results in the arrest of the bulk of the haemorrhage liable to occur from postero-lateral arteries at the prostatic rim. Considerable time is added to the operation and shock is apt to be correspondingly greater than in the previous method.

This operation is now largely superseded by that of Harris.

METHOD OF HARRIS

This method, which owes its inception to S. Harry Harris, of Sydney, was first practised by him in 1927. Essentially it consists of an immediate reconstruction of the urethra, carried out after the removal of the prostate, by suturing the apex of the trigone to the urethra above the verumontanum, and obliterating round a catheter the antero-lateral parts of the prostatic pouch.

Special instruments, e.g. illuminated retractor, boomerang needle holder, and ligature carrier are necessary for the performance of this operation which Harris has described in detail in the *British Journal of Surgery* for January 1934.

Summarizing his account he draws attention to the advantages which the method presents in:

1. Complete and immediate control of haemorrhage by suture.

2. The plastic covering of all raw surfaces in such a way that the prostatic urethra is in a great part reformed, and the prostatic cavity obliterated, with the result that healing takes place generally by first intention, septic complications are remarkable for their rarity, fistula formation does not occur, and post-operative recurrence or obstruction is completely obviated.

3. Obliteration of dead spaces.

4. The abolition of suprapubic drainage.

5. First intention healing.

Careful pre-operative treatment is necessary, particularly with reference to preliminary catheter drainage, and the verification of functional renal adequacy.

The steps of the operation, as practised by Harris, consist in:

(1) The transverse skin incision 3 in. in length, about 2 in. above the symphysis.

(2) Incision of the bladder at its highest point, with arrest of all bleeding points in bladder and abdominal wall.

(3) Bimanual intraurethral enucleation of the prostate, every attempt being made to remove the adenomatous part of the prostate without damage to the verumontanum and the anterior commissure (Fig. 30).

(4) Visualization of the prostatic cavity by means of the illuminated retractor, and the arrest of haemorrhage by the insertion of two or more haemostatic sutures at the postero-lateral angles of the prostatic cavity.

(5) Reconstruction of the floor of the prostatic urethra by the suturing of the apex of the trigone as far as possible downwards into the prostatic cavity, by means of the boomerang needle passed through the bladder wall behind the interureteric bar and made to emerge just above the verumontanum (Fig. 31).

(6) Obliteration of the prostatic cavity, and re-formation of the side walls of the new urethra by the insertion of deep anterior transverse sutures—two, or rarely three, being sufficient (Fig. 32).

(7) Insertion of a urethral catheter into the bladder, and its suspension by a silkworm gut stitch to a rod placed on the anterior abdominal wall after closure of the vesical and parietal incisions.

The urethral catheter is retained *in situ* for 10 days, irrigation being avoided unless the catheter becomes obstructed by clot.

Removal of the catheter is effected by cutting across both

DIAGRAMS REPRESENTING STAGES IN HARRIS'S OPERATION OF
PROSTATECTOMY (AFTER HARRIS).

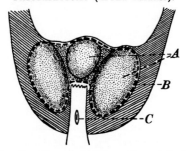

Fig. 30. Coronal section through bladder and prostate showing moderate
enlargements of lateral and middle lobes (*A*), with line of enucleation
(dotted) (*B*), and verumontanum (*C*).

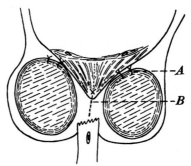

Fig. 31. Prostate enucleated. Haemostatic stitches at postero-lateral
angles of prostatic cavity (*A*). Trigone stitched into posterior wall of
cavity (*B*).

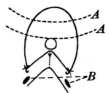

Fig. 32 *a*. View of internal urinary
meatus from above after trigonal
suture. *A*, *A*, Lines of insertion of
boomerang needle for obliteration
of anterior part of prostatic cavity.
B, Ureteric orifices.

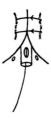

Fig. 32 *b*. Anterior stitches inserted. Catheter *in situ*,

limbs of the silkworm gut suture below the rod when the hairpin-shaped remnant is withdrawn with the catheter *per urethram*.

PERURETHRAL OPERATIONS ON THE PROSTATE

Perurethral operations on the prostate are of two types, and take the form of:

(1) Diathermy and fulguration.
(2) Resectoscopic removal.

These two methods are occasionally combined. Owing to the prevalence of post-operative suppuration in the former method, this is largely being superseded by the latter.

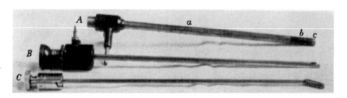

Fig. 33. Author's fulguration urethroscope. *A*: *a*, Barrel; *b*, Bakelite insulator; *c*, Terminal circular electrode. *B*, "Bundle" (light, lens system, irrigating channel). *C*, Introducer.

(1) DIATHERMY AND FULGURATION

This consists in promoting coagulation necrosis of the tissues by means of the high-frequency current, applied by an electrode introduced through the operating cysto-urethroscope, or by some specially constructed urethroscope which carries its own electrode, e.g. that of the writer (Fig. 33), acting as the positive pole. The negative electrode consists of a flat metal plate surrounded by gamgee tissue soaked in hypertonic saline, and applied to the buttock, thigh or abdominal wall.

The area of the prostate which it is desired to remove is treated with an application of the electrode until it first blanches, and later chars, with the formation of sloughs which by their separation, from 5 to 10 days later, leave a free channel for the passage of the urine. The process is carried out under visual control, the urethra being distended and kept free from blood by means of a continuous stream of water introduced through a separate channel in the urethroscope, and light being maintained by an electric bulb at the distal end coupled to a portable battery.

This process, to be satisfactory, entails three stages: first, the formation of a groove in the enlarged prostate from the immediate removal of a comparatively small amount of the prostatic tissue; secondly, the separation of sloughs, which still further enlarges the urethral channel, usually shed between the fifth and tenth day and occasionally accompanied by haemorrhage, although generally slight in amount; thirdly, a general shrinkage of the whole gland due to electro-coagulation similar to that which takes place in the treatment of vesical papillomata—previously described in chapter VIII.

As has been mentioned, this method has now few applications, but the writer has occasionally found it of value in those cases of very large soft prostate in which the actual removal of tissue by the resectoscope is insufficient, in patients who are judged unsuitable for prostatectomy. Modifications of this method are numerous, including the various "punch" methods of Kenneth Walker and Bumpus.

By means of the urethroscope (shown in Fig. 33) the whole prostatic urethra can be subjected to the action of the high-frequency current, after which the insertion of a catheter for 5 days is called for. Its removal is followed later by dilatation with a Kollmann's dilator on one or more occasions, until all sloughs have been removed and urine is passing naturally. Its chief drawback lies in the fact that the amount of tissue to be removed depends very largely on necrosis and septic separation of a comparatively unknown amount of tissue.

(2) RESECTOSCOPIC REMOVAL OF THE PROSTATE

This very valuable addition to the electro-surgery of the prostate owes its inception largely to Joseph F. McCarthy, of New York, and consists in the visual removal through an operating urethroscope of strips of the prostate by means of a wire loop acting as a positive electrode and connected with

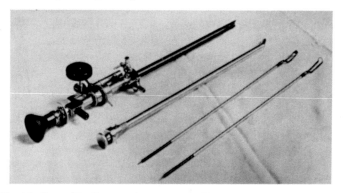

Fig. 34. Canny Ryall prostatic resectoscope, with introducer, diathermic "roller" (for arresting bleeding), and spare wire loop.

an endothermic current. This loop is activated by means of a ratchet on the proximal end of the urethroscope.

The Canny Ryall modification of the McCarthy resectoscope (shown in Fig. 34) consists of an outer sheath of bakelite of large gauge which is passed into the bladder *per urethram* with the aid of an introducer. On removal of the introducer the irrigation channel is attached by tubing to the flow of water which can be regulated by a tap on the resectoscope. The inner bundle consisting of lens system, electric light, and wire electrode, is then introduced through the bakelite sheath.

The internal urinary meatus is next inspected and the areas for removal determined. The endothermic apparatus is coupled to the wire loop with the intervention of a foot switch. By means of manipulation, both of the urethroscope and the ratchet attachment, the wire loop can be made to pass beyond the area of prostate to be removed. The stream of water is temporarily turned off and the ratchet or lever moved, so that when the current is turned on by depressing the foot switch the wire loop cuts through the prostatic prominence, retracting it into the bakelite sheath. The withdrawal of this electrode (together with light and telescope) brings to the outside the strip of tissue removed. The electrode is reinserted, the stream of water turned on, and the process repeated until sufficient tissue has been ablated.

On completion of the operation a catheter—preferably of the Eynard type—with multiple eyes is tied into the bladder for 48 hours, the removal of which usually results in the normal passage of urine. In a few cases its retention may be necessary for 5 days.

This operation is particularly indicated in cases of fibrous prostate and prostates with well-marked local intravesical prominences, in cases of carcinoma with retention where a permanent cystostomy would otherwise be necessary, and in cases in which the risk of prostatectomy would be unjustifiable.

Its chief disadvantages lie in the (comparatively) small amount of prostatic tissue removed, and inability to control the coagulating (and therefore necrosing) effects of the electrode. A too vigorous application of the instrument has occasionally resulted in the formation of fistulae into rectum and elsewhere. Bleeding is rarely severe, and can usually be controlled by the visual application of a blunt electrode to a spurting artery when seen, or by the indwelling catheter.

Chapter XIII

THE NURSING AND GENERAL MANAGEMENT
OF THE UROLOGICAL PATIENT

As in general surgery, so in urology, operation is merely an episode in the treatment of any particular disease. Nevertheless, as it is both the most spectacular, and probably the most severe incident in any course of treatment, it is a convenient pivot about which to enumerate and describe certain considerations for the management of the urological patient. Furthermore, the highly specialized nature of urology demands a careful watch, on the part of the surgeon and nursing staff, for certain signs. Unless these signs are definitely sought, they may be overlooked or not assessed at their correct value.

The following suggestions as to pre- and post-operative management may be of help to the medical man in issuing instructions to any nurse not conversant with the more recent methods of urological treatment.

GENERAL CONSIDERATIONS

Operations on any part of the urinary tract involve a greater or less strain on renal function, and attention to diet is not without value. Foods with a heavy nitrogen content should be forbidden, while fluids in the form of barley water, cherry-stalk tea, and imperial drink, should be given freely. Soups, meat and alcohol are better avoided.

Attention to the bowels is essential—a mild saline purge generally being the most helpful.

It goes without saying that the urine should be examined daily and the measure recorded, and any abnormal constituent (e.g. albumen, pus, blood or sugar) duly reported.

A separate urine chart is advisable, and where the patient is passing water *per urethram* special attention should be directed towards frequent micturition. Nor can it be too strongly impressed on the nursing staff that a marked "frequency" of only a few drachms of urine at a time is in a large proportion of cases no frequency at all, but the sign of an overflowing and distended bladder.

Symptoms of grave moment before and after operation generally result from failure—partial or total—of renal function, and may call for urgent intervention on the part of the surgeon, irrespective of the precise nature of the case. Such signs as temperature above 102° or below 97°, or rigors, together with a rapid pulse, vomiting and intense headache, drowsiness or delirium are so obvious that they would, of course, be reported to the surgeon-in-charge. On the other hand, no less important although less noticeable, are the dry, hard and brown "parrot" tongue, hiccup and thirst—particularly if associated with a diminished secretion of urine. Where thirst is a marked symptom the amount of fluid consumed should be charted against the measure of urine collected.

Urinary antiseptics in some shape or form may generally be prescribed with advantage to every case calling for operation on any part of the urinary tract.

OPERATIONS ON THE KIDNEY

Operations on the kidney take the form of drainage, removal of calculi, fixation of the kidney and removal of the kidney itself.

In those cases in which the kidney substance has been incised a certain—although perhaps not very great—liability to haemorrhage is incurred, and a watch should be kept for signs of external bleeding (if a tube has been inserted), haematuria and concealed internal haemorrhage about the kidney. Colic, from the passage of clots down the ureter, is not uncommon. Where a drainage tube has been inserted attention should be directed to the character of the discharge, and an attempt made roughly to estimate the proportions of urine and pus.

If a nephrectomy has been performed, a little blood will generally be found in the urine for the first day, but in addition to the possible complication of post-operative haemorrhage from the vessels in the severed renal pedicle, careful watch must be maintained for the functioning of the opposite kidney, and if for any reason the forcing of fluids by the mouth is impracticable, rectal or subcutaneous saline must be administered.

After nephropexy the patient should be nursed in a recumbent position for 3 weeks at least.

OPERATIONS ON THE URETER

These take the form of incision for the removal of calculi, or transplantation of their lower ends into the bowel.

Where a calculus has been removed from the ureter—whether or not that duct has been sutured and its continuity maintained—a drainage tube down to, but not into it will generally have been inserted through which small amounts of urine may be discharged for some days.

The administration by mouth of methylene-blue pills—particularly if combined with hexamine—will not only act as a mild antiseptic but will also indicate clearly the presence of a urinary discharge.

The drainage tube should not be removed before the fourth day, and then only if the discharge is small in amount and appears to be subsiding. A piece of corrugated rubber may profitably be substituted if the discharge continues.

After cystoscopic operations on the ureter, e.g. dilatation and lubrication in order to aid the passage of a calculus, all the urine passed must be carefully inspected for the presence of the stone, which may be very small and is sometimes passed with an entire absence of pain. Where the urine is thick or contains pus it may be necessary to strain it through muslin for examination of the residue.

Transplantation of the ureters is an operation of some magnitude, and, in addition to the general preparation of the patient and his urinary system, particular care must be taken with the emptying and cleansing of the lower bowel. Two or three days before operation colonic washouts should be instigated, and the administration of some intestinal antiseptic may be helpful. Charcoal is perhaps the most useful, and may be most conveniently given in the form of carboserin.

After transplantation of the ureters, singly or together, there is as a rule a marked drop in the renal output for the first 2 days. Every attempt to augment this by the oral or subcutaneous administration of fluids must be made. A special *caveat* against the administration of rectal salines in these cases is necessary, as the uretero-sigmoid junction might be imperilled by the injection of a large enema or a quantity of saline *per rectum*.

Methylene-blue pills by the mouth are a great help in announcing the first arrival of urine in the rectum, but they are not always well borne by the stomach—particularly after operation. Neotropine may sometimes be profitably substituted.

When ureteric catheters have been inserted into the ureters and brought out *per rectum*, particular watch on their drainage is called for, and at any sign of blockage they must be carefully washed out with a few c.c. of sterile saline or water. This can be most easily accomplished by means of a 5 c.c. syringe with fine nozzle attachment with a terminal eye which fits the catheter.

The measure of urine excreted by rectum or catheter should be charted. If one ureter still remains attached to the bladder, the amount of urine passed *per urethram* should be chronicled separately.

OPERATIONS ON THE BLADDER
AND PROSTATE

The bladder not only acts as a urinary reservoir, but is the area of junction of upper and lower urinary tracts. Growth or stone in its interior may call for removal by operation. It is a means of access to operations on the prostate, and cystostomy may be performed to relieve stress on the kidney when urethral obstruction exists.

Here, both before and after operation, urinary antiseptics have a more fruitful field of application than in any other part of the urinary tract. If the urine is alkaline or very foul, pyridium and neotropine are perhaps the most useful, while the various preparations of hexamine—including cystopurin and cystazol—are of little value except in an acid medium. In order to promote this condition, sodium benzoate and acid sodium phosphate are valuable, but sometimes cause diarrhoea, when their use must be discontinued.

Bladder washes may assist in overcoming a cystitis before operation, and preventing or lessening its occurrence after that event.

When continuous drainage through a cystotomy wound has been effected this should, if possible, be connected with a long sterile rubber tube discharging its contents into a Winchester at the side of the bed—the distal end of the rubber tube lying below a measured quantity of antiseptic. Every possible precaution for keeping the surrounding parts (abdominal wall, groins, scrotum, and back) absolutely dry must be taken, which will sometimes necessitate constant attention on the part of the nursing staff.

If catheter drainage is instituted the same principles should be maintained, but the urethral catheter should be changed every other day and the urethra irrigated (except after Harris's operation).

After most operations on the prostate, haemorrhage is apt

to be profuse and sometimes dangerous, while clot formation in bladder and prostatic pouch may give rise to severe pain or to blockage of the drain tubes. On rare occasions, clot formation may even necessitate the reopening of the bladder.

Post-operative urinary extravasation in these cases is fortunately nowadays rare, but if for any reason the suprapubic drainage tube becomes displaced it may occur, and should be suspected when an unaccountable rise of temperature takes place, and its presence sought about the wound, scrotum, or penis.

The patient should be protected from draughts, and be nursed in the semi-recumbent position after recovery from the anaesthetic and shock. The bladder should be washed out once or twice daily, unless the operation has been that described as the method of Harris. Particular attention must be given to the back if bed sores are to be avoided. It should be thoroughly washed with soap and water at least four-hourly, the palm of the hand being used to rub the skin and so promote the circulation. After drying thoroughly, methylated spirit should be well rubbed in and then powder (equal parts of boracic, zinc and starch) dusted over, or some ointment (e.g. zinc with castor oil) may be used in place of the spirit. The groins require attention in the form of washing with soap and water, careful drying and the application of ointment at least twice daily.

The patient should be encouraged to move himself about in bed. (If the rubber connections attached to his catheter or suprapubic tube are long enough the bed will not suffer.)

At the earliest possible moment the patient should be got out of bed into a chair, with the drainage apparatus attached. In most cases of prostatectomy, and nearly all prostatic resections, this can be effected 48 hours after operation.

The scrotum should be supported on a pillow, and at any complaint of testicular pain epididymitis should be suspected, and if present treated.

Chapter XIV

APPENDIX

The following drugs and preparations comprise a short Pharmacopoeia for use in urological cases.

A. Bladder Washes

Solution of oxycyanide of mercury, 1/8000 to 1/4000.
Solution of silver nitrate (strong astringent), 1/2000 to 1/500.
Solution of potassium permanganate, 1/4000 to 1/2000.
Solution of potassium citrate, 2 drachms to 1 pint as a preventative to blood clotting.
Hydrogen peroxide, the official solution (10 vols.) diluted 5 or 6 times and gradually increased in strength.
Boracic acid, 5 to 15 grains to 1 ounce.

B. Drugs which render the Urine acid

Ammonium chloride, 5 to 30 grains.
Acid potassium phosphate, 5 to 30 grains.
Acid sodium phosphate, 5 to 30 grains.
Benzoic acid, 5 to 15 grains.
Ammonium benzoate, 5 to 30 grains.
Salicylic acid (sodium salicylate), 5 to 20 grains.
Massive doses of sodium or potassium citrate or tartrate.
Mandelic acid, 3 grammes t.d.s., generally given with half a drachm of ammonium chloride.

C. Drugs which render the Urine alkaline

Tartrates, citrates, and carbonates of potassium, sodium, lithium, and calcium, 5 to 60 grains.

Sodium or potassium acetate, 5 to 20 grains.

D. Diuretics and Diluents

Tea, coffee, gin, barley water, imperial drink (cream of tartar, sugar, and lemon), cherry-stalk tea.

Caffeine citrate, 5 to 30 grains.

Pilocarpine (hypodermically), 1/20 to 1/2 grain.

Salyrgan [Bayer Ltd.], 0·5 to 2 c.c. intramuscularly once or twice daily. Contraindicated in cases of acute nephritis.

E. Urinary Antiseptics

Hexamine (urotropine) (hexamethylene-tetramine), 5 to 15 grains.

Hexamine and methylene-blue pills (hexamine 3 grains, methylene blue $\frac{1}{4}$ grain), 2 or 3 t.d.s.

Cystazol (hexamine benzoate in effervescent mixture) [Allen and Hanbury], 2 drachms t.d.s.

Cystopurin (hexamine sodium acetate) [Genatosan Ltd.], 30 grains t.d.s.

Cylotropin (a mixture of hexamine and sodium salicylate) [Schering Ltd.], 5 c.c. intravenously. If given intramuscularly a local anaesthetic should be used in addition.

Pyridium (a complicated preparation supplied by Menley and James), 2 tablets (equals 3 grains) t.d.s.

Neotropine (a similar type of preparation to pyridium, supplied by Schering Ltd.), 1 to 2 tablets (equals $1\frac{1}{2}$ to 3 grains) t.d.s.

Acriflavine [Boots], $\frac{1}{2}$ grain pills t.d.s.

Hexylresorcinol (caprokol), 2 to 4 capsules, each capsule containing 0·15 gramme.

F. Local Anaesthetics for Urethra

(1) Cocaine hydrochloride　gr. vi.
　　Sodium bicarbonate　　gr. vi.
　　Chloretone　　　　　　gr. iii.
　　Aq. dest. ad.　　　　　℥ iiss.
　　(Not more than 4 drachms to be used for any one patient.)
(2) Tutocain [Bayer Ltd.], 3 to 5 per cent. combined with adrenalin.
(3) Decicain [Bayer Ltd.], 1 to 2 per cent.
(4) Borocaine [B.D.H.], ½ to 2 per cent.

G. Miscellaneous

Indigo-carmine Martindale. 10 c.c. of 0·4 per cent. solution for intravenous injection.

Collargol, 5 to 10 c.c. of 5 per cent. solution for pyelolavage (½ ounce can be instilled into bladder in cases of severe cystitis).

Abrodil [Bayer Ltd.] (a stable organic solution containing 52 per cent. iodine. Not decomposed in the system). X-ray. Intravenous pyelography, 50 c.c. of 40 per cent. solution. Retrograde pyelography, 5 to 20 c.c. of 20 per cent. solution.

Solution of sodium iodide, 14 per cent. for retrograde pyelography.

K.Y. jelly [Johnson and Johnson] and Lubafax [Burroughs and Welcome], urethral lubricants. Emollient and soluble in water.

Solution of cocaine and almond oil (2 per cent. cocaine hydrochloride in equal parts of almond oil and castor oil), lubricant for ureteric calculi.

INDEX

Printed in the United States
By Bookmasters